Beautiful Skin *of* Color

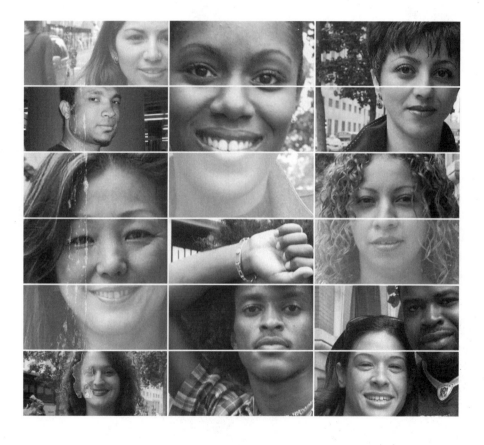

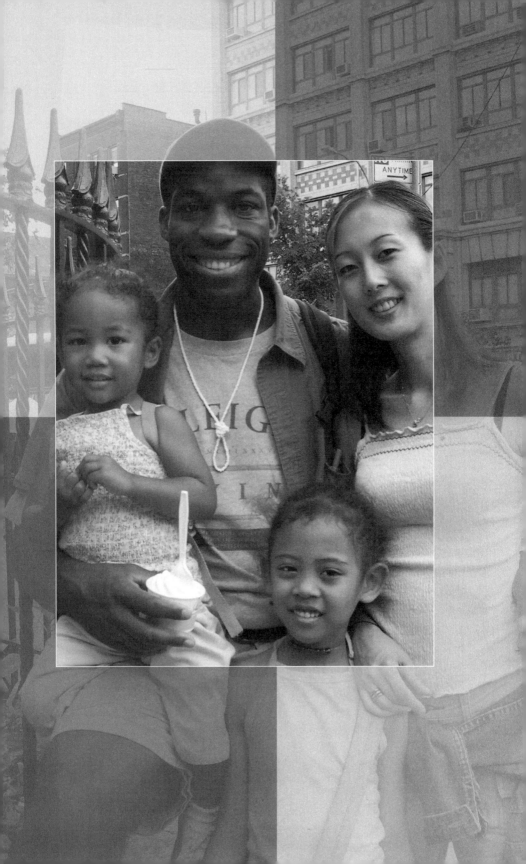

Beautiful Skin *of* Color

A COMPREHENSIVE GUIDE TO ASIAN, OLIVE, AND DARK SKIN

Jeanine Downie, M.D., and Fran Cook-Bolden, M.D.,

with Barbara Nevins Taylor

ReganBooks

An Imprint of HarperCollins*Publishers*

A hardcover edition of this book was published in 2004 by ReganBooks, an imprint of HarperCollins Publishers.

First paperback edition published 2005.

Designed by Yee Design

Photographs by Barbara Nevins Taylor and Nick Taylor

The Library of Congress has cataloged the hardcover edition as follows:
Downie, Jeanine.
    Beautiful skin of color: a comprehensive guide to Asian, olive, and dark skin/Jeanine Downie and Fran Cook-Bolden; with Barbara Nevins Taylor—1st ed.
      p. cm.
    ISBN 0-06-052153-8 (alk. paper)
    1. Skin—Care and hygiene. 2. Beauty, Personal. 3. Minorities—Health and hygiene.
  I. Cook-Bolden, Fran. II. Nevins Taylor, Barbara. III. Title.

RL87.D69 2003
646.7´26´089–dc22

2003061068

ISBN 0-06-052155-4 (pbk.)

05 06 07 08 09 ❖/RRD 10 9 8 7 6 5 4 3 2 1

For our families:

Michael Bolden, Natalie, Michael (Mikey), and Alfred (Al);
Michael Heningburg, Jr., and Jade;
and Nick Taylor.
You are our everything.

Contents

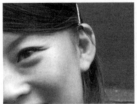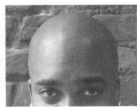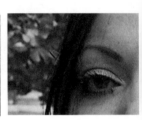

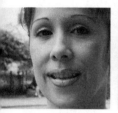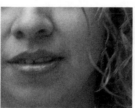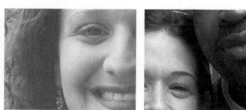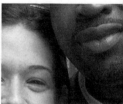

Introduction

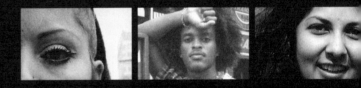

CONSIDER *Beautiful Skin of Color* YOUR PERSONAL SKIN CARE HAND-book. If your family has roots in Africa, Asia, the Caribbean, Latin America, the Indian subcontinent, the Middle East, the Mediter-ranean, or the South Pacific or is Native American, *Beautiful Skin of Color* unlocks the particular secrets of your skin and provides the answers you've been searching for. You deserve them.

Beautiful, healthy skin and great hair are within your reach. Whether you're a woman or a man, we know that your skin and hair speak for you. Your appearance influences the way you feel about yourself. When you look good, you feel good. It's one of the funny things about life. You feel more confident when your skin glows and is free of blemishes, and your hair is healthy, manageable, and stylish. It's easier to go to school or work, to clean the house, to go on a date, or to take on the world. Your attitude about life changes.

And that's why we wrote *Beautiful Skin of Color.* We want to give you the knowledge and the information you need to look your best.

We know from our personal experience that very little accurate information is available about Asian, olive, and dark skin. It's frustrat-ing. People whisper about persistent acne, or the dark marks that appear frequently on the skin, or ingrown hairs and unsightly bumps on the back of the neck. Well-meaning people often make recommen-dations to try to solve the problems without really knowing the full story, and that can be dangerous. Many problems arise in Asian, olive, and dark skin because of misinformation, inadequate care, or improper treatment.

You may be too shy to talk about your skin, or it may seem too personal to share your problem with others. You may have searched in vain for a medical professional who is knowledgeable about skin of color. We know that it often seems like no one understands. We hear you, and we want to help.

As you read *Beautiful Skin of Color* you'll find letters and e-mail from real people who share your concerns. They are just like you. They, too, are searching for answers.

In each chapter, we tell you the real story about your skin. We tell you why you have skin of color, and why your skin is olive, or dark, or very dark. We hope that you look for answers on every page. We also hope that you'll read *Beautiful Skin of Color* from start to finish, but we have organized this handbook alphabetically, so you can turn to sections as you need them. Each chapter provides specific information about various medical and cosmetic issues. We explain why they happen and suggest remedies. We offer suggestions about what you can do on your own, and what you should expect when you seek a doctor for guidance.

Skin Management

As you read *Beautiful Skin of Color*, think of yourself as the manager of your skin. We find that most skin issues are management problems, and we make practical recommendations to help you manage and improve your skin.

By using the information in each chapter, including the listings of selected products that we find effective, you can set up simple, new routines to follow every day. We'll give you explanations that will help you decide when it is wise to see a doctor. And after visiting a doctor, you can incorporate the doctor's recommendations with a solid at-home skin management program.

Throughout *Beautiful Skin of Color* we talk repeatedly about skin management and other topics that we think are important. Please don't get impatient with us. Some things bear repeating.

The need for sun protection is a theme that runs throughout *Beautiful Skin of Color*. We like the sun. But we don't like sun damage. No matter how dark your skin, or how you've treated it in the past, we hope that you will begin to use sun protection immediately. We describe the importance of sun protection in almost every chapter and also devote an entire chapter to this subject.

We are concerned about the way you, and others, handle your skin. Asian, olive, and dark skin tends to be supersensitive. And we remind you in every chapter to treat your skin *gently*. Whether you have acne or dark marks or want to improve your appearance with chemical peels, Botox, wrinkle fillers, laser treatments, or one of the new technological advances we describe, it is essential to make sure that you, and the professional who treats you, handle your skin *gently*.

There's one more thing. Having beautiful skin and hair can make you happy, and happiness, in return, can make your skin and hair beautiful and healthy. We hope that you enjoy yourself as you read *Beautiful Skin of Color*, and that you smile occasionally as you see your-self and the solutions to your problems in the pages of this book. Happy reading.

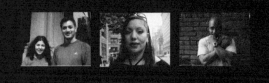

About Your Skin

CHAPTER 1

WE LIVE IN A SKIN-COLOR-SENSITIVE UNIVERSE. MOST OF US ARE keenly aware of variations in our complexions and in the skin of others.

How many times have you wondered, "Why is my skin this color?" How many times have you asked silently, "Why is my skin different?" These are really good questions. Too often, the answers are political or filled with some kind of rhetoric that has nothing to do with the basic questions.

The real answers about skin of color are deeply embedded in the very essence of your being. Skin of color has a unique cellular makeup and a special protein structure. The cells and the skin structure create and replenish the beautiful color. They also make the skin particularly susceptible to damage. There's a paradox. Although dark skin is delicate, the darker pigment protects the skin, to some degree, from the damaging ultraviolet rays of the sun.

Your skin reacts the way it does for various reasons. Everything that happens on the surface of the skin reflects something going on inside your body.

One guiding force determines everything. It is the most significant piece of our biological puzzle. It is DNA—the genetic pattern that you inherited from your parents. DNA is embedded in the nucleus of every one of your cells. In each cell, it acts like a set of instructions providing a blueprint for the way you are supposed to look.

When you smile and see your mother's grin, or suddenly notice

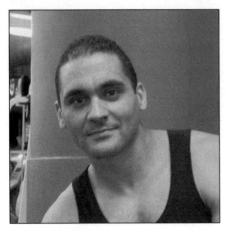

that your eyes are like your father's, you've spotted the work of DNA. DNA carries the message that makes you who you are.

The message is transmitted at the moment of conception. When a sperm fertilizes an egg, cells divide and chromosomes are created. These chromosomes containing your parents' DNA develop in the nucleus of your cells. The instructions, of course, aren't all the same. There are separate sets of instructions, transmitted through about two hundred different types of cells to all parts of your body.

The skin is the largest organ of the body, with its own special cells. There are 30 million cells in one square inch of your cheek; each cell contains the plan for the way your skin will look. The instructions come to you from your parents, grandparents, great-grandparents, and an ancient family tree linking you to men and women who lived thousands of years ago.

The work of researchers in a number of fields is helping us learn more about our genetic lineage. An important discovery came after anthropologists found the remains of a man buried in the ice of the Italian Alps. They nicknamed him Siberian Man and established that he had been buried for five thousand years. In 1994, Oxford University professor Bryan Sykes traced Siberian Man's DNA. Professor Sykes determined that Siberian Man's DNA matched the DNA of Europeans who are alive today. This significant piece of scientific detective work has enormous relevance for us as we try to understand ourselves and the difference in skin of color.

Certainly, the physical appearances of men and women have

changed over the centuries as we adapted and shape-shifted to meet the demands of nature and our cultures. It's unlikely that you'll find a look-alike for Siberian Man in Europe today. But there are people who share his DNA, and somewhere in their body chemistry or physical makeup, something of the five-thousand-year-old man lingers.

There's plenty of research, and a great deal of speculation, about how different cultures evolved. We're not going to jump into that. But if your family history includes people from Africa, Asia, the Caribbean, the Indian subcontinent, Latin America, the Mediterranean including Greece and Italy, and anywhere in the Middle East, Turkey, or the South Pacific, or if you are Native American, you have genes and cells that react similarly to genes in the darkest skin of color.

You are in a world of company. Imagine creating a world map and identifying all the countries where people with skin of color live. White patches would include only European countries, Russia, Australia, Canada, and the United States. Even that is changing. The 2000 United States Census revealed a significant increase in the number of people with skin of color in the United States, and the report predicted that number will grow. People with skin of color—African-Americans, Asians, and Latinos—may account for half of the population in the United States as we move into the twenty-first century.

The statistics support trends we see in our daily lives. Skin color differences in the United States and elsewhere are blurring because of immigration and the marriage of cultures. Similarly, immigration is changing Europe's population. Cultures are blending, and faces are changing there, too.

The slow melding of cultures has occurred over the centuries. African-Americans and Caribbean-Americans dragged from their homelands as slaves often had little choice as to who would father their children. Native Americans and Latin Americans were frequently subsumed by rulers who changed the genetic patterns of their offspring. Of course, people also happily and willingly intermarried, creating new patterns of DNA.

There are very public examples. Academy Award–winning actress Halle Berry's mother is white, and her father is African-American. Tiger Woods's mother is from Thailand, and his father is African-American. The Rock, the popular wrestler and actor, has a family history blending the DNA of his mom from Samoa, in the South Pacific, with his dad's African-American heritage.

In Thailand, Cindy Burbidge is a beautiful television host and model, and a former Miss Thailand. Her father is American, and her mother is Thai. With her blue eyes and fair skin, people question whether or not she's actually got any Thai blood. Cindy asked the rhetorical question of a New York Times reporter, "How can you prove that you're Thai? How can you prove that you're anything?" Cindy's mom, her dad, and her DNA provide the answer.

Many, without hard facts and information, can't trace their family history. Yet people you've never known, and never imagined, have had something to do with the way you look. Mixed ancestry may explain why people in the same family often have different shades of skin color. Yet the person in the family with the lightest skin is likely to share the skin sensitivities of the relative with the darkest complexion. The DNA in cells contains the historical tale and a distinct plan. It makes skin of color, regardless of the shade, much more sensitive and reactive than white skin.

Our Dominican-American friend Carlos appears to have milky-white skin. His dad and mom have olive skin. "Although I'm really light-skinned," he says, "I still get dark marks on my face after I get a pimple." Carlos develops dark marks because his DNA says he has skin of color. When his skin is traumatized by acne, his fair skin reacts like skin of color and produces dark marks.

Skin of color is particularly reactive because of its cell formation and the way its protein works.

How the Skin Works

Your skin is like a rich layer cake with amazing things filling every layer. The surface is a remarkable outer garment that serves as a protective barrier, warding off bacteria, the environment, chemicals, poisons, and the pushes and pulls of everyday life. The skin filters water and prevents you from getting waterlogged. It also helps to keep the water you need inside your body. Sweat glands in the skin regulate temperature. You sweat to cool off when you're too hot, and you get chills, or goose bumps, when you're too cold. Nerve receptors in your skin talk to you all of the time. They signal the tingling feeling at the moment of a sensual caress and make you flinch or groan when you're pinched or hit. Muscles deep in your skin cause tiny hairs to stand on end when you're frightened or aroused. What goes on below the surface determines the reaction on the surface, including the color.

Epidermis

The top layer of skin, called the *epidermis,* is actually made up of fifteen to forty layers. The number of layers of the epidermis depends on the area of the body. The skin is thinnest under the eye and on the eyelid. It's much thicker on the sole of your foot. The overall thickness depends on your sex and your age. In most places, the skin thins as you get older.

You may be surprised to know that most of your surface skin is made up of dead cells. Most of the epidermis is a collection of flattened, protein-filled cells stacked on top of each other. As the cells move from one layer to the next, they produce filaments of a protein called *keratin* as well as a granular substance called *keratohyaline.* The grains and the filaments clump together and gradually kill the cells during a process called *keratinization.* These are the same type of cells that make up your hair and nails, although the skin on your body is much softer and more flexible.

By the time they get to the surface, these keratinocyte cells are tough guys. They've produced proteins that bind them together. And they've created their own lamination to waterproof the skin and protect it against bacteria, chemicals, light, and heat waves. If you look under a microscope, or if your skin gets very dry, you can see the way the hexagonal cells connect to one another. But the cellular connection is usually so smooth that you rarely notice.

You also rarely see the skin shedding. But every four to five weeks your skin renews itself and the old cells become dust. You may shed as many as two pounds of dead skin cells every year. The process is seamless because new cells replace the old immediately. These new cells appear fresh as they reach the surface; they haven't been battered by the environment or the wear and tear of rubbing and pulling.

This constant renewal is healthy and actually can improve your appearance. In the chapters that follow we explain how you can speed up the natural process to stimulate new surface cells.

The epidermis also contains Merkel or nerve cells that send sensory messages through receptors to the brain, Langherans cells that help to fight disease, and melanocyte cells that are at the core of the color issue.

The Cellular Difference

Melanocyte cells produce the pigment, or *melanin,* in your skin. Everyone, regardless of his or her color, has the same number of melanocytes.

Melanocyte cells produce tiny packages of granules called *melanosomes.* The melanosomes are a superexpress color delivery system working twenty-four hours a day, seven days a week. Each melanocyte cell is clear with a dark spot in the center and has a network of arms extending outward. These arms deliver the melanosomes, or packages of color, to the surrounding keratinocyte cells. And the keratinocyte cells carry the pigment to the surface to give your skin and your hair color.

> **FACT:** *Melanocyte cells produce tiny packages of granules called* melanosomes. *The melanosomes are a superexpress color delivery system working twenty-four hours a day, seven days a week.*

The actual color is determined by a few factors. There are two primary types of melanin produced by the melanocytes: eumelanin and pheomelanin. People who have Asian, olive, and dark skin produce more eumelanin than people with fair skin. And people with fair skin produce more pheomelanin than people who are darker. Your DNA determines the type of melanin your cells produce.

There are other significant differences. The size and placement of the melanosomes, those packages of color created by the melanocytes, are a crucial part of the reason your skin looks the way it does. The pattern of melanosomes is different in people of color. Melanosomes are large and spread out in dark skin. In white skin, they are smaller and more densely packed.

Different ethnic groups appear to have different-sized melanosomes. A recent study that compared the melanosomes of African-Americans, Mexicans, Indians, and Chinese found that African-Americans had the largest melanosomes. Indians had the second largest. Mexicans had the third largest, and the Chinese study participants had the fourth largest melanosomes. All of these ethnic groups had larger melanosomes than Europeans.

This is an important cellular distinction. But there is more. The melanocytes in dark skin are very active. They are busy all of the time. Your melanocytes produce more pigment than melanocytes in white skin. The precise amount of color depends on your DNA, the genetic instructions in your cells. In all skin, melanin helps to protect against the sun's ultraviolet rays. And that's one of the functions of pigment.

Another important factor makes your skin special. People with skin of color also have a unique protein structure. That structure is at work below the epidermis in the *dermis*.

Dermis

The dermis also has layers, and it varies in thickness throughout your body. The dermis is filled with a network of blood vessels, hair follicles, nerve fibers, muscle cells, sweat glands, oil glands called *sebaceous glands*, bundles of protein fibers called *collagen* that give the skin strength, and elastic fibers that allow the skin to stretch. Collagen bundles together and with the elastic fibers creates a latticelike framework for your skin cells. The collagen-elastin support system is the source of firmness, fullness, and elasticity. Wrinkles begin in this layer of skin when the collagen and elastin wear out. In Asian, olive, and dark skin the structure of collagen explains why your skin reacts differently to stresses than white skin does.

The Protein Difference

Collagen protein is made up of amino acids. The amino acids are arranged in a specific sequence predetermined by your DNA. In skin of color, the collagen is bundled together more thickly than it is in white skin. If you are African-American or Asian, or have olive skin, you may have heard that your skin is thicker than white skin. That's not quite right. The thick bundles of collagen simply give dark skin a different physical tone.

There is a great deal about skin of color that we don't know. And many questions can't yet be answered. But scientists are continuing to investigate issues involving skin of color, including the cellular and structural differences. It is important to find answers because they will help us treat medical conditions like *keloids*—thick scars that grow larger than the original wound. Keloids are particular to skin of color.

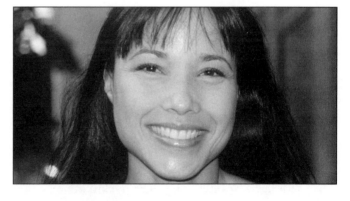

For now, though, it's useful to take a look at the rest of the skin, which functions the same way, for the most part, in everyone.

The hair follicles in the dermis are made of keratin. These tiny hairs are invisible in many places. They are everywhere on your body, except on the palms of your hands and the soles of your feet, and a few other areas.

If you have bouts of acne or oily skin, these hair follicles play a big role. The hair follicles are connected to the sebaceous glands, which produce the oil that pops up on the surface of your skin. When there's oil on the skin, acne isn't far behind. We explain how acne develops in chapter 2.

The dermis also helps to regulate your body temperature. It is the home of the sweat glands. These are called the *eccrine glands*. You have millions of these sweat glands all over your body. They're trying to maintain a steady temperature inside. When your body is too hot, or when you're stressed or eat spicy food, these glands produce a salty solution that evaporates on the surface to cool you off.

Blood vessels in the dermis are part of the heat regulatory system. When the outside temperature is hot, or when you're nervous and the heat builds up inside of you, your skin gets a little red. Those tiny blood vessels are helping out. They're dilating to get rid of the heat. In the cold, the blood vessels constrict to hold in the heat.

And last, and we wish they were least, we have another set of sweat glands in the dermis. The *apocrine glands* produce body odor and ear wax. These are holdovers from the days when we needed to use our natural scent to attract the opposite sex.

Subcutaneous Tissue

The bottom layer of skin is called the *subcutaneous tissue*. There's a thick collection of collagen and elastin in the subcutaneous tissue. This gives the skin a strong and stable base. Again, the collagen protein has a different structure in skin of color. The collagen in this layer of skin of color is also denser and collected in thicker bundles than it is in white skin.

You may not like it, but everybody needs some fat. We come prepackaged with it. Your fat layer is in the subcutaneous tissue. You need the padding for your bones and other organs. The fat layer also provides insulation. When you're hungry, and don't have time to eat, it provides a little energy to keep you going. The subcutaneous tissue also produces the vitamin D required to keep our bones healthy.

The Bottom Line

Your skin is a special and complete system. It is easily damaged and requires special care. Read on!

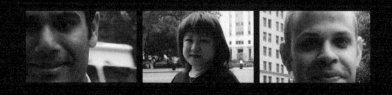

Acne

CHAPTER 2

ACNE IN ASIAN, OLIVE, AND DARK SKIN CAN REALLY MAKE YOU FEEL AS though you've lost control of your body. And in a way, you have. Even the mildest case of acne is a serious problem for skin of color. The tiniest blemish unleashes a chain of events that's difficult to combat.

It is a case of one bad thing following another. First you spot a pimple. The pimple goes away. And instead of clear skin, you can bet you'll have a dark mark. These dark marks are important reasons to pay immediate attention to acne breakouts. We know that *all* skin of color is sensitive, and Dr. Henry W. Lim of Henry Ford Hospital in Detroit finds that Asian skin is particularly vulnerable. "When Asian skin gets acne, it tends to be more severe."

Acne is a personal issue for us.

"I'm passionate about treating acne," Dr. Downie says. "When I was about twelve, I started getting these annoying little pimples on my forehead. I grew my hair out to cover my forehead. And then suddenly, I had pimples all over my face. I hated it. And of course my brothers made me feel worse because they teased me. They called me 'Pizza Face.'"

Dr. Downie was lucky. Her acne calmed down in her twenties. Dr. Cook-Bolden didn't have acne when she was younger and thought she'd go through life without it. Then her body surprised her.

"I never had acne as a teenager. Now that I'm a grown-up, with three children, I wake up some mornings and I'm confronted with acne breakouts on my face. It's embarrassing. I'm the dermatologist, and even though I know better, I think this isn't supposed to happen," Dr. Cook-Bolden says.

Acne is humbling. It doesn't matter who you are. Although the breakouts are beyond your control and it is important to understand that there is no cure for acne, it is possible to manage it. Tackling the problem by yourself is difficult. There's a confusing array of products on store shelves. When we're shopping in the drugstore, we frequently notice people struggling to decode the labels on the acne remedies, and we often want to stop and help.

When we received Angel's e-mail, we thought she spoke for millions of other acne sufferers: "I've been breaking out since I was thirteen. It started on my forehead. My mom always said it would go away. I'm nineteen years old now and the problem is worse. I have tried everything I can get my hands on. Nothing seems to work. I have a lot of marks from old breakouts. They make my face look worse. I never go out without makeup. This is really a big problem. It brings down my self-esteem. Why is this happening?"

Why It Happens

You've heard people question whether eating habits contribute to acne. A small percentage of people develop acne as a result of what they eat. Fried foods or chocolate may cause acne flare-ups in some people. For most people, however, food does *not* trigger acne. Yet in every case, a healthy diet including fish, grains, green vegetables, fruits, fiber, and water can help to improve your skin.

People also incorrectly assume that dirty skin causes acne. Cleanliness is always important, but cleanliness does not prevent acne.

Acne is primarily caused by what happens inside your body.

Your hormonal system gets acne going. You're likely to have the first flare-up at the beginning of adolescence when your hormones kick in. Angel experienced that, and so did Dr. Downie. It's why children between eight and thirteen years old are suddenly humiliated by eruptions on the face, and sometimes on the neck, back, chest, and buttocks. Acne is one of the things that makes adolescence really tough.

FACT: *Fried foods or chocolate may cause acne flare-ups in some people. For most people, however, food does* not *trigger acne. Yet in every case, a healthy diet including fish, grains, green vegetables, fruits, fiber, and water can help to improve your skin.*

The Androgen Factor

You probably have heard about the hormone androgen, which you may automatically connect to men. Although men produce larger quantities, women produce androgen, too. Your glands begin to manufacture androgen when you are an adolescent. You see the effect as hair grows under your arms and in the pubic region. When acne bumps begin to form, it's another sign that your body's chemistry is changing.

If you're acne-prone, androgen may enlarge the sebaceous glands that are deep in your skin. These oil-producing glands are connected to tiny hair follicles that you can't see. The follicles open at the pores, which are tiny holes on the surface of the skin. When everything is healthy and works properly, the oil naturally lubricates your skin. But when androgen gets overactive, you have a problem.

The androgen stimulates the sebaceous glands to pump out more oil. And the oil interacts with the bacteria that we all have on, and in, our skin. The excess oil clogs up your pores with the formation called a *plug*. Clogged pores trap the bacteria that naturally lurks in the hair follicles under the skin. With nowhere to go, the bacteria gets agitated. It causes inflammation and redness. It produces chemicals and enzymes that spew out fatty acids. Now the clogged pores are really stopped up.

Acne appears in two forms: noninflammatory acne and inflammatory acne.

Noninflammatory Acne

If you develop *noninflammatory acne*, you're likely to see blackheads or whiteheads on the surface of the skin. When you have a blackhead, it means that the hair follicle is open. It isn't a speck of dirt inside the hole. The air from the outside has seeped into the open pore and darkened the oil. You're actually looking at a tiny spot of discolored oil.

If you have a whitehead, it means that your pore is closed. The oil hasn't been exposed to the outside air, and it hasn't been discolored. But underneath that closed pore is a buildup of oil pressing against the surface of the skin.

Inflammatory Acne

The first signs of *inflammatory acne* are swelling and inflammation. This looks and feels quite different from blackheads and whiteheads. You have inflammatory acne when you see bumps and blemishes on the surface of your skin. You're also likely to have deeper, swollen, and tender or even painful bumps under the skin. When inflammatory acne forms, there's a lot of activity going on underneath the surface. Pressure builds up under the skin. Clogged pores burst. White blood cells are stimulated. And boom—you have larger pimples, redness, swelling, pus, and cysts along with blackheads and whiteheads. It is possible that you'll have severe inflammation. If you don't get treatment, the inflammation can cause deep scars.

In skin of color the line between noninflammatory and inflammatory acne may be blurry. Researchers found that when people of color get a blackhead or whitehead, the skin is often inflamed. This is another reason why it's important to get the proper treatment.

Natural Healing

At some point your immune system kicks in and the anti-inflammatory process begins. The acne can heal on its own. But it may take days, weeks, or even months. For some people, it may take years. It all depends on your body. With skin of color, as the acne heals, the dark marks appear.

If you treat the acne, you can shorten the process and control the discoloration. Again, if you have inflammatory acne, nothing you do on your own is going to help significantly. It's important to seek treatment and develop a management plan with your doctor.

When Angel's mother predicted her acne would go away, she was partly right. Often, hormones quiet down a little bit when you're in your twenties. But you don't truly outgrow it, as Shelly describes in her e-mail: "I'm twenty-nine years old now, and my acne hasn't gone away. It is so embarrassing. It stops for a while and starts up again. My skin has a mind of its own. Nothing stops the acne."

We wish that we could say that the acne will go away tomorrow. We can't. If

> **FACT:** *At some point your immune system kicks in and the anti-inflammatory process begins. The acne can heal on its own. But it may take days, weeks, or even months. For some people, it may take years. It all depends on your body.*

you are acne-prone, you are likely to have persistent flare-ups throughout your life. But you can manage the acne and the dark marks. You can take control and prevent the acne from getting worse.

Dr. Cook-Bolden says, "You will always have hormones, and your hormones will always fluctuate. They're affected by many things, including stress and biological factors."

In a way, acne does have a mind of its own. It may have been built into your system before you were born. Some researchers believe it is a matter of genetics. They think acne is preprogrammed in the DNA in our skin cells. There's also a theory that if you are predisposed to acne, stress triggers hormone activity and pumps up the androgen level.

The Difference Between Men and Women

Although acne attacks men and women equally, men tend to have more severe cases because of the androgen factor. Men produce more androgen, and when the androgen is overstimulated, it can create the type of acne that leaves deep scars. It starts early in a young man's life. Valerie wrote to us about her son: "My fourteen-year-old son has dark skin and is very handsome. For the last few months, he has had a bout of terrible acne on his forehead and on his back. I'm afraid that it will leave scars."

Valerie's right to be concerned. The cellular and protein makeup of skin of color makes it extremely sensitive. An adolescent, young, or middle-aged man who has a severe acne breakout is at risk of developing serious scars.

Nathaniel is an adult struggling with the problem: "I'm a thirty-six-year-old male with acne. It is really bad on my forehead. I can't seem to get my skin to smooth out. When I'm at work, I can swear that everybody is looking at my acne. Sometimes, I won't look at people who are talking to me because I can keep the conversation short by not making eye contact. When I'm in the sun my acne is magnified ten times, which makes my face even worse. HELP!"

Severe acne involves body chemistry and is beyond your individual control, although it can be managed with the guidance of a knowledgeable doctor. People with mild cases of acne, perhaps a few pimples, don't necessarily need to visit a dermatologist, but it is essential to get treatment for serious acne. It is extremely important for men whose hormones are actively pumping out androgen and overstimulating the sebaceous glands.

Aggressive treatment at the beginning of a severe acne cycle is the best way to contain acne and prevent serious scarring.

Hormones and Female Adult Acne

Being female didn't protect you from raging androgens when you were a teenager, and your gender will not protect you as you mature.

Women naturally produce androgen in their ovaries and adrenal glands. If your body makes a lot of androgen, you're likely to break out. Your female hormones, the estrogens, can help you. Your menstrual cycle causes changes in your estrogen and progesterone levels. Acne sometimes gets better when you have your period, but it's more likely to get worse because the hormone levels are changing.

Estrogen can be helpful, and your doctor may prescribe it, in the form of a birth control pill, to counter the androgens.

Hormonal changes during pregnancy also have an effect. If you're pregnant and you've always had clear skin, you may begin to break out. Or if you've struggled with acne for years, you may find that your skin clears up during pregnancy. The extra estrogen and progesterone you are producing create the swing.

Remedies

What You Can Do on Your Own

First, recognize that you have acne. "Most people come into my office with dark marks. That's what they focus on. They want to cure the dark marks right away," Dr. Cook-Bolden says. "But I tell them that they have to control the breakouts in order to stop the dark marks."

TIP: *Once you recognize that you have acne, you can begin to manage it. We think a few changes may be needed in your daily routine. You can control mild cases of acne without visiting a doctor, and it is worth the effort.*

It's possible that you may not even realize that you have acne. Acne breakouts in skin of color can be gray, purple, or brown, while they are often pink or red in lighter skin. Dr. Downie says, "People think that their acne is a rash, fungus, or cancer. When I tell them that they have acne, they disagree with me. They say, it's not like the acne that I see on TV, or on my white friends."

Once you recognize that you have acne, you can begin to manage it. We think a few changes may be needed in your daily routine. You can control mild cases of acne without visiting a doctor, and it is worth the effort.

Control Oily Skin

Even if you don't have acne, your skin produces oil. If you're acne-prone, you want to reduce the oil that feeds the acne on your face and all other areas of your body where acne appears. Oil should not be in any product that you put on your skin, including makeup, shaving cream, and sunscreen. Oil is the enemy. Products containing oil block the pores and feed the pimples.

Some widely used beauty products can make acne worse. For

example, many people use cocoa butter and other greasy products to smooth the skin. These products contribute to acne. In addition, hair sprays that contain an oily sheen invariably are sprayed on the skin and clog the pores.

Check out the fine print. Don't be fooled. Even if the package says "oil-free," it doesn't necessarily mean it's right for you. The product may contain other ingredients that are greasy and will clog the pores and stimulate acne. Look for products with labels that say "non-comedogenic," which means it doesn't clog the pores, or "nonacnegenic," which means it doesn't stimulate acne. Some labels may even say that the product "doesn't clog pores." It's a good idea to test a product by placing a small amount on your forehead to see how it feels.

> TIP: *Check out the fine print. Don't be fooled. Even if the package says "oil-free," it doesn't necessarily mean it's right for you.*

For Women: Bobbi Brown, I-Iman Makeup, Shiseido, Neutrogena, Prescriptives, and MAC are among the companies that make oil-free makeup for a range of skin tones. Neutrogena's makeup even contains an antiacne agent.

For Men: We like Aveeno Shave Gel and Razor Defense Shave Gel by Neutrogena. They are both thick, rich gels that help prevent irritation.

Cleansers

Neutrogena Oil-Free Acne Wash and Cetaphil are good basic cleansers for everyday use. Washing your face, or the parts of your body affected by acne, once in the morning and again in the evening may not be enough.

Make friends with your skin. Look at it. See what it is telling you.

You may need to wash more frequently to reduce the oily buildup. Neutrogena Alcohol-Free Toner is a mild astringent that will remove flaky skin. We also like Oxy soap and cream for cleansing extremely oily skin. Salac foam and products that contain benzoyl peroxide and salicylic acid are also effective because they kill bacteria, help to dry the skin, and open clogged pores.

> **IMPORTANT:** *Make friends with your skin. Look at it. See what it is telling you. You may need to wash more frequently to reduce the oily buildup.*

Many products are packaged under drugstore or generic brand names, and they can be useful for milder cases of acne. Proactiv is an over-the-counter product that contains a step-by-step plan. If your acne isn't severe, and you follow the program, it can make a difference.

Keep in mind, however, that not everyone's skin reacts the same way to every product. It is a good idea to experiment a little bit. Try one product at a time to see which works best for you.

Alpha and Beta Hydroxy Products

Alpha and beta hydroxy acids were originally nature's gifts to the skin. Over the centuries clever people have used a variety of plant-, fruit-, and food-based acids to renew and enhance the skin's texture. Applying acid to the skin at first sounds frightening, and most chemical acids will hurt. But alpha and beta hydroxy acids are miraculously beneficial when used in the proper, diluted amounts and applied correctly.

Alpha and beta hydroxy acids can help unplug clogged pores, smooth skin tone, even out color, improve texture, and minimize fine lines and wrinkles without causing long-term damage because they work with your body's chemistry. The top layer of skin is a collection of dead cells that slough off every four weeks to five weeks. You rarely notice the process because old cells are quickly replaced by cells that haven't been beaten up by the environment.

Alpha and beta hydroxy acids speed shedding by helping to break the bonds that hold the surface skin cells together. The acids also increase cell production and help to seal in moisture. In addition, they stimulate the body's natural collagen, which plumps out fine lines and gives the skin a nice texture. We recommend using cleaners, toners, wipes, moisturizers, and peels that contain alpha or beta hydroxy acids. In most cases, after regular, consistent applications your skin will look fresher, brighter, and healthier.

Many alpha hydroxy products contain glycolic acid, which was originally derived from sugar cane. Lactic acid is another widely used alpha hydroxy acid, and it was originally made from milk. Beta hydroxy acid, or salicylic acid, is naturally found in the bark of the white willow tree and the wintergreen plant. Natural acids are still available. But most alpha and beta hydroxy products on the market contain a synthetic version of the acids that is equally effective.

Doctors use alpha and beta hydroxy acids in varying formulations in their offices to treat acne. Over-the-counter products are a good place to start if you are not seeing a doctor. They are milder and have a lower percentage of acid in their formulations than those sold by prescription or in a dermatologist's office.

Many cleansers contain glycolic acid. For Asian, olive, and dark skin we like Aqua Glycolic, and a product called Alpha Hydrox that comes in a bright red box. Avon Anew, also one of our favorites, is readily available via the Internet or through an Avon representative. Facial Cleanser by NeoStrata is a gentle cleanser with gluconolactone, a special formulation of alpha hydroxy acid, which helps to improve skin tone. These are reasonably priced products that are easily accessible and contain an amount of glycolic acid that is safe to use without a doctor's supervision.

Beta hydroxy acid, or salicylic acid, is good for very oily skin because its anti-inflammatory agents help to slow excessive oil production.

Neutrogena Oil-Free Acne Wash and Neutrogena Clear Pore Treatment, which can be applied at night, contain beta hydroxy acid. Oxy Balance deep cleansing shower gel for both face and body is a beta hydroxy product, and there are also drugstore generic brands that include beta hydroxy acid.

Some cleansers are packaged as wipes or are individually wrapped. It's a good idea to carry them with you to use when your skin feels greasy.

Dermatologists sell cleansers manufactured by companies like M.D. Forte, Refinity, Glytone, and Glyderm. These products have higher concentrations of the hydroxy acids and because they're stronger, they usually work better. They are, however, slightly more expensive. Whatever you use, we recommend setting up a daily routine to apply the alpha or beta hydroxy acids either in the morning or the evening.

One thing to watch out for: the hydroxy acids may make your skin too sensitive to allow eyebrow or facial waxing. And it very important to wear a sunblock with a sun protection factor (SPF) of 20 to 30, preferably with titanium oxide or zinc oxide.

If your skin is too sensitive for alpha and beta hydroxy acids, the formulation in NeoStrata's products containing gluconolactone seems to be gentler.

Gently Does It

Whatever you use, remember the word *gently*.

Gently wash your face and the affected areas. Don't scrub or rub. Rubbing makes the acne worse. Avoid rough scrubs and loofah mitts. They tear the skin and are likely to cause irritation and create dark blotches.

Avoid Picking

It is hard to keep your hands away from your face when you'd like to squeeze a pimple or a blackhead. But this is harmful. Squeezing, picking, and poking make more trouble. You traumatize the skin and increase the inflammation. The dark marks and indentations that form after picking are often harder to treat than the acne. Picking is a sure way to damage your skin. We can't say it louder or clearer.

Over-the-Counter Remedies

There are effective over-the-counter creams, lotions, gels, and pads to go along with the cleansers. They often enhance each other and enable you to establish an acne-fighting routine. Again, it is important for you to look at your skin and do a little self-analysis. If your skin is sensitive, creams and lotions are generally better for you. People with normal and oily skin can use a liquid or a gel. But gels and liquids contain alcohol and may dry out the skin too much. It's best to use gels only on very oily areas of your skin. For mild cases of acne we like Clearasil and Neutrogena On-the-Spot Acne Treatment, Neutrogena Alcohol-Free toner, and products containing benzoyl peroxide, which by drying out the skin, can help to fight the bacteria that clogs pores and makes acne worse. If you have very oily skin, Clinac O.C. is an excellent over-the-counter product. It is applied after you wash your face and can help reduce the oil.

Sun Protection

The sun loves pigment. It stimulates the melanocytes—the pigment cells that give you your skin color. And those cells are already overactive. The acne has already turned them on. You may say, "I'm dark. I don't burn." It doesn't matter how dark you are. You need an oil-free, noncomedogenic sun protection that contains Parsol 1789, UVA and

UVB protection, and a sun protection factor of between 20 and 30, preferably with titanium dioxide or zinc oxide. We explain what all of this means in the sun protection chapter.

Beyond Basics

We've described basic things that everyone can do for pimples and mild cases of acne. But if the acne is more severe and persists, it is a good idea to visit a board-certified dermatologist who understands Asian, olive, and dark skin. Shop for a doctor as you would for a pair of shoes or a household appliance. Ask questions. Does the doctor have patients who look like you? If you can, ask those patients if they are satisfied with the treatment they are getting. Take the time to make sure that you get the best doctor for you. Not everyone is familiar with treating skin of color.

A Doctor's Guidance

"This is really a partnership," Dr. Cook-Bolden says. "In order to treat your acne, you have to make a commitment to follow through and to use the doctor's recommendations. I tell patients, 'I can help you. But if you don't do your part, my part is not going to work.'"

Your doctor will evaluate the acne, and depending on the severity, recommend a combination of therapies.

"There is no magic pill," Dr. Downie says. "But acne treatments are so much better now than they were when I was a teenager. We can make a huge difference, if you work with us."

The goal is to reduce oil production, clean up bacteria, clear the clogged pores, and quiet down the inflammation and the redness. Doctors like antibacterial and anti-inflammatory creams to soothe the inflammation and often prescribe these creams in combination with a retinoid, which is a prescription-strength vitamin A cream. Studies show that vitamin A, like the alpha and beta hydroxy acids, stimulates the skin's natural collagen and improves the tone and texture of the skin.

While the retinoid is working on the skin texture, it is also unclogging the pores. When the pores are open, the antibacterial creams can get in to do their work. Remember when you use a retinoid or any other medication, more is not better. A tiny pea-size amount spread on the affected area is enough. If you use too much, your skin will get very flaky and red. Although the irritation will subside in a few days, it is better not to overdo it. Some people experience excessive flakiness and peeling even when they do everything right. This reaction generally stops after repeated use. Among the retinoids that a doctor might prescribe are Retin-A Micro, Tazorac Cream, Avita Cream, or Differin Cream.

Your doctor may also prescribe oral antibiotics to decrease the inflammation of acne. These antibiotics might include: tetracycline, minocycline, or doxycycline; antibiotics in the cephalosporin family like Keflex or Ceclor; or an erythromycin like EES tablets. Antibiotics are generally safe and can be good medicinal tools. But it is important to be aware of the potential side effects.

Let your doctor know if you've had allergic reactions to antibiotics. We don't recommend antibiotics for pregnant women. Antibiotics can reduce the potency of birth control pills. They may cause severe vaginal yeast infections in women who are prone to these infections. Studies have found that a small percentage of those who take antibiotics suffer from upset stomachs, dizziness, and bluish discoloration of the skin. Antibiotics also make the skin sensitive to the sun. Children under ten should never take tetracycline; it can discolor their teeth.

If you can tolerate the antibiotics, however, they are very useful.

Chemical Peels

We talked about the alpha and beta hydroxy acids in the products you can use at home. Alpha and beta hydroxy acids are the central ingredients in chemical peels used in the dermatologist's office, and when they are applied by a knowledgeable doctor, they are far more effective than any of the over-the-counter preparations. Chemical peels are part of our new arsenal of skin rejuvenation techniques. They are an important part of acne treatment because they prepare the skin and allow topical medications to penetrate more deeply. Peels also help to unclog the pores, smooth the skin, fade the dark marks, and even out the skin tone. A doctor is likely to recommend a series of chemical peels as part of an acne management program. One peel may be helpful, but you'll need several to really see a difference.

Warning

There is an important warning: If you have had herpes, let your doctor know before the peel. The herpes virus lives on nerve endings in the skin. If a cold sore is not completely healed, a chemical peel may activate the virus. The doctor will prescribe medication that can prevent a flare-up.

The Peel

The strength and type of peel will depend on your skin. Typically doctors use glycolic acid, salicylic acid, lactic acid, or trichloroacetic acid. Doctors frequently make custom combinations of alpha and beta hydroxy acids to fit your skin type and achieve better results. For Asian, olive, and darker skin, we again say, go *gently*.

You want to improve your skin without doing damage. It is too easy to overstimulate the pigment cells and create dark spots and blotches. The wrong kind of peel administered by the wrong person can seriously damage the skin.

Understanding the way the peels work may help.

The higher the acidic content in the peel, the more irritating it is to the skin. Peels range from 20 percent of acid in the solution to 99 percent. A peel with 20 percent solution is unlikely to be irritating, or to redden the skin. You should be able to go back to work immediately. These light, superficial solutions are often called "lunchtime peels."

Moderate and strong peels may keep you out of work or in the house for a week or more. When these peels are applied the skin becomes tight and dark and peels in sheets. The skin is red and often raw.

We recommend superficial to moderate peels for Asian, olive, and darker skin.

You can't be too careful about choosing the person who administers the peel. State laws often restrict the acid content that can be used by nondoctors. But because Asian, olive, and darker skin is highly sensitive, the mildest peel may damage your skin.

Even in the doctor's office, start with a mild peel. Typically it would have an acid content of between 20 and 35 percent. Some people will graduate to a 70 or even a 90 percent acid solution peel. The doctor should monitor you carefully. Everyone's tolerance level is different.

And it's important for you to communicate with the doctor. When we administer a peel, we ask you to tell us on a scale of one to ten how much your face burns or tingles. We do not want you to get up to ten. It is possible the solution will remain on your skin for five minutes or longer. Some doctors apply a neutralizer or ask you to rinse your face with cool water immediately when the time is up. We generally recommend six to twelve peels administered every two to four weeks so there is minimal irritation.

Chemical peels make the skin sensitive. It is important to apply an appropriate sunblock. Your skin may be too sensitive for facial or eyebrow waxing for a few days after the peel. The wax can easily burn the skin. And immediately after a peel, take care to avoid kissing or rubbing against someone with a herpes or a fever blister for at least a week. The virus can attach itself to the newly peeled skin and cause scarring.

COST

The cost of a chemical peel can vary widely—from $125 to $2,000 depending on the depth of the peel. Doctors may negotiate a package rate for a series of peels that will reduce the overall cost.

Severe Acne

Severe acne means that you have cysts and nodules, or big bumps, deep in your skin. They are usually very painful. The cysts are those deep, pus-filled, inflamed spots that can cause scarring.

If you have severe acne, your doctor is likely to prescribe an oral medication such as Accutane or a generic version of the drug whose chemical name is isotretinoin. Two of these drugs are marketed under the names Amnesteen and Ranbaxy, although there is some question about whether the generic drugs are as effective as Accutane. If you take Accutane faithfully as prescribed and follow the rules, it works.

Doctors have been prescribing Accutane since 1982, when it was approved by the FDA for the treatment of severe cystic acne. Eighty-five to 90 percent of patients who take Accutane find that it clears their acne. Treatment usually lasts about five months, but it could take several years to clear up your skin. Accutane must be taken under a doctor's supervision. There are strict guidelines for prescribing and using the drug. Your doctor will perform blood tests before you begin, and then will monitor your blood every month throughout the treatment, because there can be significant side effects. In addition, you will be given a medication guide and required to sign an informed consent form.

Accutane can cause birth defects, and pregnant women shouldn't use it. Health officials worry about young women who use the drug, ignore the rules, and become pregnant. They've asked doctors to issue stern warnings. If you've used Accutane in the past, ask your doctor when it's safe to get pregnant. Other possible side effects include dry eyes, dry mouth, nosebleeds, muscle aches, and poor night vision as well an increase in the level of bad cholesterol and liver damage. There is also concern that Accutane causes depression and could lead a person to have suicidal thoughts.

Despite the possible side effects, many patients use Accutane and don't have any major problems. This is important because without the help of a drug like Accutane, it is very difficult to get some cases of acne under control.

Accutane is most effective when it is part of an overall skin management program. Your personal program created with your doctor's help should include an at-home care regimen. The combination of medication and consistent care speeds the skin's renewal and can help you to conquer the acne.

Cortisone Injections

Cortisone is part of the group of medicines known as corticosteroids. Doctors use cortisone for a wide range of problems, including acne, allergic conditions, respiratory problems, inflammatory arthritis, and even certain types of cancer, because it often effectively reduces inflammation. We use cortisone injections to help flatten raised scars, and if your acne is very bad, and your bumps are large and inflamed, your doctor may inject cortisone directly into the pimple. The injections do two things: they flatten the pimple, and they help to prevent scarring. Sometimes when pimples shrink, small depressions are left in the skin. Cortisone may increase that possibility. Eventually, in most cases, the depressions fill in naturally.

Although the injections are often useful, we don't recommend topical cortisone to treat acne. If cortisone is used incorrectly, it can thin the skin, create broken blood vessels, cause severe discoloration and additional acne breakouts.

New Technology

Rapidly changing technology and continuing research offer creative new techniques for treating acne. Laser, light therapies, and perhaps radio frequency waves have the potential to revolutionize the way acne is treated. Some doctors are using laser and light systems to control and slow down moderate acne breakouts, and they often use these techniques alone or to supplement other types of treatment. After a consultation and evaluation your doctor will help you to determine if one of these methods should be included in your acne treatment plan.

THE GOOD NEWS: *In recent years, lasers and other light sources have been developed that are safe for use on skin of color.*

Doctors call laser, light, and new technological treatments *nonablative*—meaning the devices do not cut, burn, or harm the surface of the skin. The procedures work by producing effects deep in the layers of the skin.

In recent years, lasers and other light sources have been developed that are safe for use on skin of color. Now researchers report promising results about laser and light treatments that reduce oil production and bacteria. Although doctors aren't certain about all the reasons why laser treatments are having this effect, it is helpful to understand how the laser works.

Laser Treatment

Laser stands for *l*ight *a*mplification by *s*timulated *e*mission of *r*adiation. The laser creates energy in the form of a single beam of light or, as scientists call it, a coherent beam of light. The energy can be used in a variety of ways by altering the length and the intensity of the beam. To treat acne the beam is directed to pass through the outer layers of the skin. The laser's energy targets the sebocytes, the oil-producing part of the sebaceous glands.

Researchers think the heat from the laser shrinks the sebaceous glands, resulting in decreased oil production and bacteria. This is significant because when you reduce the oil production, you slow one of the triggers for acne. In addition, the laser light also seems to stimulate chemicals in the immune system called *cytokines,* which act as anti-inflammatory agents.

The laser treatments also help renew your skin's natural collagen, which can improve skin texture and reduce some scarring and dark marks.

At the time of a laser treatment, the doctor will ask you to wear protective eyewear. The doctor may apply a cooling gel, and it's possible that you'll feel a rubber-band-like snap or stinging as the doctor treats the area. The treatment may take five to fifteen minutes. Some redness or swelling might develop, but you should be able to return to your normal activities immediately.

The number of treatments will vary with the severity of the acne. It is possible that you'll need only one. If you have severe acne, you may require two to four treatments during a four-week period for six months to a year.

The price of the treatments will vary depending on the skill of the doctor and where you live. Treatments for individual laser sessions generally range from $300 to $500. Doctors are likely to work out package prices for multiple sessions.

Light Treatment

Light treatments are similar to laser treatments, but the light sources do not use a single focused beam of energy. Researchers discovered that high-intensity light penetrating the skin stimulates molecules called *porphyrins,* which are produced naturally by acne bacteria. The porphyrins become confused and create oxygen that kills the bacteria.

Although the technology is new, the idea behind the treatment is not. Until scientists determined the connection between the sun's rays and skin cancer, doctors frequently asked patients to sit under sunlamps to dry out acne bumps. The new light treatments eliminate the harmful rays.

Not all doctors are convinced that light treatments are an effective way to treat acne. But doctors who are researching these techniques are enthusiastic about the results. Several types of light systems are being studied. Some doctors are currently using pulsed light treatments and a system called ClearLight.

PULSED LIGHT TREATMENT

Pulsed light treatments are administered with a handheld instrument regulated by a computer that directs intense pulsed light directly at specific areas of the skin.

CLEARLIGHT

ClearLight is the name of a system developed by Lumenis that uses an intense narrow band of blue light to target acne. Doctors are typically using ClearLight to treat acne on the face, neck, chest, and back. The FDA has approved this treatment for mild and moderate cases of inflammatory acne.

THE DOCTOR'S PROCEDURE

When you receive a light treatment, the doctor will ask you to wear eye protection. A doctor may use a gel or a cream to numb the skin. During pulsed light treatment you may feel a light rubber-band-like snapping as the light hits the skin. You're unlikely to feel any discomfort when you are treated with the ClearLight system.

The light treatment may last from five to thirty minutes. Your skin may be slightly pink after a treatment, but it should clear quickly. The number of treatments will vary depending on your skin type. If you are having intense pulsed light or ClearLight treatment, your doctor may recommend eight treatments over a four-week period. Doctors who use the ClearLight system recommend two treatments a week for eight weeks.

·After a series of light treatments it may be four months before another treatment is required.

COST

Treatment costs will very depending on where you live and on the system that's used. Prices could range from $50 to $400 per session, and doctors are likely to create a package price for multiple sessions.

Radio Frequency Waves

Using energy created by radio frequency waves to stimulate collagen and new cell production is another innovation that's being tested for acne treatment. We describe how radio frequency wave treatment works in chapter 24 on skin rejuvenation. Researchers theorize that the heat from the frequency waves damages the sebaceous glands and reduces the amount of oil that's produced. They believe the treatment may be beneficial for people who suffer from moderate acne. Research is still in the early stages, and it is not clear whether radio frequency wave treatment is a viable option for treating acne.

COST

A radio frequency wave treatment is likely to cost between $1,500 and $2,500.

Photodynamic Therapy

Some researchers are taking laser and light therapy one step further in a procedure they call *photodynamic therapy*. They are investigating combination therapies involving laser or light treatment and a solution called Levulan that is applied to the skin before the laser or light treatment and, in some cases, seems to enhance the work of the light source.

Levulan is approved by the FDA for treating precancerous skin conditions. During these treatments doctors discovered that the combination of Levulan and light improved the skin's texture. Additional studies found that Levulan appears to shrink the sebaceous glands and reduce oil.

Levulan makes the skin extremely sensitive to light and the sun. It is important to wear protective clothing, sunglasses, and sun protection for forty-eight hours after the treatment. Levulan is not approved by the FDA for acne treatment, and we think more research is required.

Acne Scarring

Scars do follow serious acne. And Pablo knows the problem. He wrote to us: "I'm a thirty-one-year-old Latino guy who needs help. I've suffered from acne since I was 18 years old. Now I have deep acne pits on my face. People call me 'Pizza Face,' and sometimes, I close myself in a room and cry."

Dr. Downie has been there. "Remember, my brothers called me Pizza Face. A dermatologist helped me get my acne under control. And that's the reason I decided to become a dermatologist. I wanted to help other people just like I was helped," she says.

If your acne has progressed and you have scars, there are several things a good dermatologist can do. And again, we caution that it is important to seek the advice of a board-certified dermatologist who understands skin of color.

Very bad acne scars are difficult, if not impossible, to clear up completely. But you can make significant improvements in your appearance. While a skilled doctor can help you, it is important to be realistic. Please don't expect baby-smooth skin.

New Technology

In some cases, laser and light treatments have been effective in reducing acne scarring. Laser treatments, in particular, are used to stimulate and renew the body's natural collagen. Some studies indicate that light treatments may also have the same effect and help to smooth and renew the skin. The treatments are based on the same principles that we described a little earlier in the chapter. A full description of the effectiveness of these treatments for skin renewal is in chapter 24, "Laser, Light, and Radio Frequency Skin Rejuvenation."

Other Treatments

Punch Grafting and Excision

Doctors call the deep holes that acne causes "Ice Pick Scars." They can be very upsetting because women find it difficult to cover them with makeup, and men can't hide them. A few surgical techniques are available that can help without damaging your skin. A qualified dermatologist can graft skin from another part of your body to fill the small holes. Dermatologists call this *punch grafting.*

The procedure is performed in the doctor's office. The doctor will use a local anesthetic. A small piece of healthy skin is removed from behind your ear with a biopsy instrument that looks a little like a hole puncher. The doctor then removes the acne-scarred skin and places the healthy skin into the opening. The area is held together with sterile surgical strips. Typically a doctor will perform two to five of these grafts during one session.

The skin should be moderately smoother, and a doctor may treat you with a nonablative laser to improve the texture even more.

When a doctor performs *punch excision,* the acne scar is removed. There is no transplant or graft. After the skin is removed, the doctor stitches or tapes the normal skin together. In a few days the area begins to heal naturally. There's very little scarring, although you may see a small mark.

These procedures are generally safe for skin of color unless there is a history of thick scarring or keloids in your family.

Dermabrasion

If you decide to explore dermabrasion, make sure that you consult a doctor with a lot of experience. Dermabrasion is usually an effective treatment for people with lighter skin. This skin resurfacing can help to treat acne, wrinkles, and scars.

Dermabrasion is like sanding the skin. First the doctor numbs the area with an anesthetic or freezing agent. The dermabrasion tool is a handheld instrument with a stiff brush attached to a rotary motor, and as the doctor moves the instrument across your face, layers of skin are removed.

As the skin is removed, the body's natural collagen is stimulated and begins to renew itself. When dermabrasion is effective, the new skin is likely to be fresher, healthier, and fuller looking because of the collagen restoration.

It can be beneficial for some skin types, but for some Asian, olive, and dark skin, dermabrasion may be too rough. It is likely to overstimulate the pigment cells and create permanent dark marks and blotches. We don't usually recommend dermabrasion for skin of color, and when we do we only like to see it performed by a skilled physician.

COST
Dermabrasion generally costs between $1,500 and $2,500.

Microdermabrasion

Suki asked, "I'm an Asian woman with acne marks and some scars. Is it safe to have microdermabrasion? Will it help clear up my skin?"

A series of microdermabrasion treatments along with other treatments that we've outlined in this chapter may help. Microdermabrasion is gentler and safer than dermabrasion for Asian, olive, and dark skin. Layers of skin are not rubbed off, and you won't need an anesthetic. Because your skin will be gently "blasted" with fine particles, you'll be asked to wear protective eyewear to prevent the fine particles from damaging your eyes. The doctor will use a handheld instrument to spray tiny crystals of salt or aluminum oxide at the area being treated. The debris and the top layer of skin is swooped up with a vacuumlike action. This is a very superficial procedure, but it also stimulates collagen production and refreshes the skin.

The process takes between ten and twenty minutes. It's likely to leave you with some redness, which should fade in a couple of hours. Your skin will be more sensitive than usual and it is important to use sunblock with UVA, UVB, Parsol 1789, and a sun protection factor of between 20 and 30, with zinc oxide or titanium dioxide if possible.

COST

Microdermabrasion generally costs between $150 and $250 per session. Doctors are likely to arrange package rates for multiple sessions to reduce the overall cost.

Laser Resurfacing

Laser skin resurfacing is another procedure that has gained popularity. The laser removes several layers of the skin, leaving you pink and raw. Laser resurfacing is not usually a good idea for people with Asian, olive, and dark skin because there's the chance that the laser's energy may overstimulate the pigment cells and create difficult-to-remove dark marks and blotches.

As we explained earlier, nonablative treatments are used effectively for skin of color when the technology is used to stimulate effects underneath the top layers of skin. New technology can be beneficial for Asian, olive, and dark skin. We'll have additional explanations about safe laser, light, and other technological advances in the chapters that follow.

Combination Treatment

Dr. Cook-Bolden says, "A combination of therapies can be very beneficial in the treatment of acne scarring. I find microdermabrasion even more effective when it is immediately followed by a nonablative laser resurfacing treatment the same day."

COST

A combination treatment of microdermabrasion and nonablative laser resurfacing may cost $350 to $1,000.

The Bottom Line

Whatever you do to treat acne and get it under control, patience and consistency are very important. Do not pick at your acne. Keep your skin free of oil, and use medication according to the instructions. You can't speed the process. It takes time. Using more medication is not better. When used incorrectly, even the best remedy can cause redness, irritation, and excessive dryness. Similarly, buying a variety of products and applying them at one time won't help. Instead, adopt a management plan that's realistic for you to follow.

Please don't give up, stop midway, or get discouraged. It may be tempting to bounce from doctor to doctor as you search for a quick fix. There are no miracle cures.

Whether you use over-the-counter preparations or prescription medicines, it may take as long as eight weeks or more to see improvement. Hang in there even if the acne persists. You can make a difference, and while the acne may not disappear forever, you can control it.

Ashy Skin

CHAPTER 3

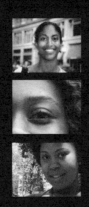

IF YOU ARE AFRICAN-AMERICAN OR CARIBBEAN-AMERICAN, YOU WERE probably a toddler when you first heard your mother say, "Oh, baby, your skin is so *ashy*. Let me put something on it." We've heard the term *ashy skin* forever. For many, ashy skin is an everyday occurrence, particularly during the dry, cold winter months. Although ashy skin isn't life-threatening, it can make you uncomfortable, itchy, and self-conscious.

Michele writes: "I'm a dark-skinned person, and ever since I was a little girl there have been flaky patches of white skin on my arms. I've tried everything and nothing I do seems to make the ashy look go away. I'm always covering up my arms."

Ashy skin is a very common problem. Dr. Cook-Bolden says, "I have very dry skin, and I have been fighting it all of my life. It can be very uncomfortable and itchy. I have to pay attention and manage it carefully. And I'm always looking for inventive ways to help my three children who are struggling with ashy skin."

Why It Happens

Basically, ashy skin is dry skin. It occurs when your skin doesn't have enough natural water to keep it moist and supple. Thirty percent of the epidermis, the outer layers of your skin, is made up of water. Researchers believe we start losing moisture in our skin as soon as we're born. As we age, we lose a little of the oil in our skin that helps to seal in the water. The sun, the wind, dry heat, irritating soaps and detergents, and diseases like diabetes also work to deplete both the oil and the water. On top of all of this, your genes—DNA—may determine whether you'll have ashy skin.

Your skin is like your garden; it is happier and healthier when it is regularly tended.

When the skin loses a lot of moisture, it gets rough and flaky. On dark skin, the flaky dry skin stands out. It looks gray and ashy. It is as simple as that. You can get ashy skin on your face and any other part of your body. But we see it most commonly on elbows, lower legs, feet, knees, and backs.

For the most part controlling ashy skin is straightforward. Your skin attracts water when it's humid. That's why it feels soft when you're at the beach, a swimming pool, or a lake, and even when there's a warm rain. Your skin is like your garden; it is happier and healthier when it is regularly tended. Skin feels wonderful and supple when it is moisturized, and you want to do everything possible to attract moisture and keep it in.

Remedies
What You Can Do on Your Own

This is one of the areas of skin management where you can be extremely effective. You can manage ashy skin, with a little effort. A basic change in the way you wash and moisturize your skin and wash your clothes can make all the difference. Establishing a new routine will help banish those ashes to the dustbin.

Controlling Ashy Skin

Moisturizing lotions, creams, and soaps are getting better all the time. Researchers are learning why certain things have positive effects on the skin, and they are experimenting constantly. Fortunately, this research is quickly translated into the development of new products.

Moisturizers work by creating a barrier on top of your skin. The barrier helps to hold in moisture. At the same time, the moisturizer creates a slight swelling effect on the surface, making the skin look smoother and healthier.

There's a wide range of moisturizers, and some are more effective than others for individual skin types. It's a good idea to try a number of products until you find the one that works best for you. There's a caution here: try one a day. Don't try them all at once.

Look for unscented and alcohol-free moisturizers. Alcohol and perfume are drying, and can be irritating.

The formulation of moisturizers is important. Moisturizing lotions are water-in-oil combinations. Ointments and heavier creams tend to be oil-in-water formulations. Cetaphil, Lubriderm, Eucerin, and Curel are good all-purpose moisturizing lotions. Creams are heavier and may feel greasier, but they are often more effective for ashy and very dry skin. Eucerin Original Moisturizing Cream, Carmol 20, Vanicream, and SBR Lipocream are preparations that can help.

Products with humectants, substances that actually attract water to the skin, are excellent. When you read the labels of the moisturizers, look for products that include either glycerin, urea, hyaluronic acid, or dimethicone.

We particularly like moisturizers that contain alpha and beta hydroxy acids. They are also humectants and enhance the work of the moisturizer as they speed shedding of dead skin cells and renew natural collagen. We recommend Jergens Ash Relief Moisturizer, Lacti-Care, LAC-HYDRIN, AmLactin, and Eucerin Renewal Alpha Hydroxy Moisturizer, which has the added benefit of a sunscreen with an SPF of 15.

The way that you use the moisturizer makes a difference. It's a good idea to apply moisturizer after a shower or bath while the skin is still damp. Lather it all over your body. Dr. Downie says, "Don't be timid. Buy a rubber kitchen spatula and use it to help you get to the hard-to-reach spots on your back. Put the moisturizer on the spatula and reach over your shoulder, or behind your back, to rub it in."

If ashy skin is persistent, use your regular moisturizer along with a little Vaseline Petroleum Jelly, lanolin, or one of the thicker creams. It may feel greasy. But these products work by forming a thick protective coating on the outside of the skin. It's like having a Band-Aid on the skin.

Acne Awareness

If you are prone to acne flare-ups, Dr. Cook-Bolden warns, "Make sure that you choose a moisturizer that says it is noncomedogenic, nonacnegenic, or doesn't clog pores. Heavy petroleum-based moisturizers will clog pores and create the climate for acne."

> IMPORTANT: *If you are prone to acne flare-ups, Dr. Cook-Bolden warns, "Make sure that you choose a moisturizer that says it is noncomedogenic, nonacnegenic, or doesn't clog pores.*

Elbows and Knees

Many people have extremely dry skin on their elbows and knees. Regular moisturizing is important for these areas. Sometimes you need to take an extra measure. You can use Vaseline Petroleum Jelly at night. It is greasy, but it provides a protective coating to seal in your own moisture.

To shield your clothes and your bedding from the grease, Dr. Downie suggests a method she's perfected for herself. "Try cutting the toes out of a couple of pairs of tube socks. After you put on the Vaseline, pull the socks over your knees and elbows," she says.

You don't have to do this every night. Try it when your skin is very ashy and itchy, or once or twice a week during the winter months to prevent the ashiness from returning.

The soaps you use and the way you wash can make a difference. Scented soaps tend to dry out the skin. We prefer unscented soaps with a moisturizing formulation. Try Dove or Oil of Olay.

Water temperature is important. Very hot water dries out the skin. Quick showers in lukewarm water are better for ashy skin than long, steaming hot showers.

If you crave a relaxing bath, fill the tub with moderately warm water and avoid scented bubble baths. Instead try soaking in Aveeno Oatmeal Bath and baby oil for about fifteen minutes. The Aveeno products have very gentle ingredients and aren't likely to irritate your skin.

Avoid Scratching

Scratching and rubbing ashy and dry skin are definite no-no's. You can easily irritate your skin and create dark marks. Maintaining short nails is an easy way to ensure that you don't irritate your skin, if you do scratch.

A Doctor's Guidance

When nothing seems to work and you're miserable, it's a good idea to seek out a board-certified dermatologist. The doctor will review your skin care routine and make recommendations that can help.

Sometimes over-the-counter moisturizers aren't strong enough. You may need prescription moisturizers.

Prescription Medicines

Your dermatologist might prescribe a strong LAC-HYDRIN 12% cream or Carmol 40. They contain strong formulations of lactic acid and help to lock in natural moisture. The stronger acid content, available through prescription, makes the moisturizer more potent.

Water

We mentioned earlier that caring for your skin is a bit like tending your garden. Your garden likes plenty of water and so does your skin. You can't pour it on, but you can drink it. Drinking water is important; it hydrates your skin and helps combat the ashiness. Dr. Downie drinks fifteen glasses of water a day, and she recommends that most people drink at least eight glasses of water.

It also helps to keep a humidifier in the bedroom in order to add moisture to the air. The additional moisture can help to make your skin, hair, and nails look and feel better.

Dr. Cook-Bolden uses a cool-mist humidifier at home for her children. She also recommends placing shallow pans of water near radiators to moisten the air throughout the house.

Detergents

Detergents get your clothes clean, but they often leave a lingering fragrance that can irritate your skin and contribute to the dryness. Fragrance-free detergents are the best for people with dry skin. All Free and Cheer Free are widely available fragrance-free detergents.

The Bottom Line

Your skin requires attention and consistent management to control ashiness. Those of us with dry skin can't neglect a regular moisturizing routine, and we must constantly replenish the moisture. It's helpful to carry a small tube of moisturizer. Keep one at your desk and your sink so that you are always prepared when your skin signals for help.

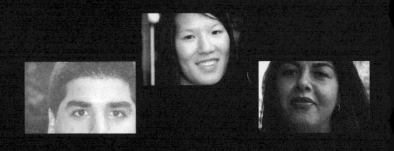

Botox

EVERY TIME WE SMILE, SQUINT, OR FROWN, WE WORK THE MUSCLES that create facial lines, making them more pronounced. These lines develop their own groove in an inevitable process that begins when we are very young. How many times did your mother say, "Don't frown. Your face will freeze like that"? Now you may be sorry that you ignored her.

Some consider wrinkles marks of character. But many of us would like to have a little less character and far fewer wrinkles. If you have very dark skin, if you're African-American, Caribbean-American, or from the Indian subcontinent, you're likely to have fewer fine wrinkles. The pigment in your skin generally protects you from the sun damage that creates wrinkles as we age. Yet if you have other types of olive and dark skin, fine lines may still be inevitable.

In any type of skin, pigment doesn't protect you from creating your own expression lines. Facial movement creates deep lines in skin of every color. "The factor is the muscle movement, and you can develop these deep lines at a very young age," Dr. Cook-Bolden says.

Alan, an African-American dentist with dark skin, had a deep groove on his forehead and a crease above the bridge of his nose. "Maybe they're occupational worry lines. Maybe I'm just a tense guy. But I wish I didn't have them. They make me look older than I am," he says.

Alan visited Dr. Downie. "Alan's typical of many patients who want to have Botox. Most people want to look younger, and in many cases they can," she says. Dr. Downie smoothed the lines using Botox.

A week after the injections, Alan called to say, "You made my wish come true. I look younger."

Despite all of the publicity and the information about Botox, many people are still uncertain. Alanthra wanted to take advantage of the cosmetic advances to improve her appearance but was a little nervous about it: "I'm a forty-five-year-old Latina with a mixed background. I have a deep wrinkle between my eyebrows. I overheard my four-year-old daughter's friend ask, 'What's that crack on your mommy's face?' I think it's time to make the crack disappear. Is it safe to use Botox?"

We think Botox is safe, and so does the United States Food and Drug Administration. Dermatologists and plastic surgeons have been using Botox to treat wrinkles since the early 1980s. It is only recently that the FDA gave Allergan, the pharmaceutical company that trademarked the name and manufactures Botox, permission to advertise it as a remedy for certain wrinkles. There is also a similar product called Myobloc from Elan Pharmaceuticals and another called Dysport from Ipsen, a British company. But Botox has become the most recognized name for the botulinum toxin that paralyzes muscles and smooths wrinkles.

How It Works

There are seven types of botulinum toxin. Botox is the brand name for botulinum toxin Type A from Allergan. Dysport is also an A toxin, and Myobloc is the brand name for a product with botulinum toxin B.

Although these are the same bacterial toxins that cause the fatal food poisoning called botulism, it's not that scary. The use of the toxin is controlled. In medical and cosmetic applications, very small, diluted amounts of the toxin are increasingly being put to good use in innovative ways. There's solid history of investigation and experimentation.

Research into the possibility of harnessing botulinum toxin A for medical use began in the late nineteenth century. In the 1960s Alan B. Scott, M.D., was trying to find a way to treat severe eye muscle twitches and crossed eyes. He discovered that when he injected botulinum toxin A into a muscle, it attached itself to nerve endings and blocked the signals that cause muscles to contract. The temporary paralysis calmed twitching and helped to realign eye muscles. Scott's research ultimately led to the development of the product now called Botox, and in 1989 the FDA approved Botox to treat eye muscles.

Doctors treating patients for eye spasms with small amounts of Botox noticed that wrinkles around the eyes and brow smoothed out. There's a simple explanation: facial expression lines are caused by muscle tension under the skin. When the muscles contract, they wrinkle the skin. It's the muscle contraction that causes the deep furrows between your brows, the lines on your forehead, squint lines, and crow's feet. Skin that can't move won't wrinkle. After a Botox treatment, shallow lines seem to fade away for three to four months.

> **FACT:** *Facial expression lines are caused by muscle tension under the skin.*

Many doctors used Botox to treat wrinkles years before it was approved by the FDA for cosmetic use. Currently, some doctors are using Myobloc, although the FDA hasn't yet approved it for wrinkles. The FDA gave Mybloc clearance in 2000 for the treatment of neck muscle spasms.

Myobloc has certain advantages for doctors. Unlike Botox it doesn't have to be stored in a freezer; it can be stored in a refrigerator. It is a prepared solution that doesn't require dilution.

There are other differences: it takes seven to ten days to see results with Botox and the effects last for three to four months. Myobloc works within a day or two, but it doesn't last as long as Botox. It wears off in two months, rather than three or four.

Both Myobloc and Dysport are widely available in Europe. Since manufacturers hope to win FDA approval, both products are undergoing clinical testing in the United States.

All of the botulinum toxin products are administered the same way. At this point, we prefer Botox. We have achieved excellent results with it, and we'll focus primarily on the way Botox is used.

Where It Works Best

The injections make forehead lines and creases between the eyebrows recede. They are also effective for squint lines, crow's-feet, and sometimes the fine lines underneath your eyes. We also like to use Botox to ease the fine lines around the mouth. Botox can effectively correct a drooping smile and even out facial expressions.

There is also hope for the aging neck without plastic surgery. You may be able to take off that scarf or put away that turtleneck. In some cases, we use Botox to reduce the horizontal lines and relax the vertical muscle bands that make a neck look old.

How It Is Administered

Injections are given in a doctor's office while you are sitting up. The doctor may ask you to squint or furrow your brow so that he or she can mark the spots that will be injected. Usually, you won't need an anesthetic. If you are sensitive, you may want your doctor to apply a topical anesthetic cream like EMLA to numb the area before the injection. Some doctors apply ice packs for numbing. The injections sting slightly. Typically, it will take three to five injections during one session to smooth the frown line between the brows. Forehead lines may require five to six injections.

The treatment is usually completed in less than ten minutes. After the injections some doctors apply ice to reduce the possibility of swelling.

Initially, there may be slight bruising and swelling, which is likely to subside in a few hours. You may be able to reduce the possibility of side effects by avoiding agents that thin your blood. Don't take aspirin or drink alcohol forty-eight hours before you receive the injections. If you are taking prescription medication such as Coumadin, which thins the blood, or herbal remedies that are blood thinners, it is likely that you will experience some bruising. These marks should fade within several days.

Some people experience a slight headache or nausea after the injections. These reactions usually go away in a few hours. Sometimes this discomfort lasts a day or two. If the problems persist, it is important to call your doctor.

WHEN YOU SEE RESULTS

If you use Myobloc, lines recede in a day or two. Botox works more gradually, and it's likely that you'll see the results in seven to ten days.

A Doctor's Guidance

The Skill of the Doctor

The doctor's skill is important. The doctor must understand facial and neck anatomy as well as the way muscles work. The injections stop the muscle action, and unless your doctor skillfully administers them, you might not be able to move your eyebrows, and it's possible your expression may seem frozen. These injections can improve your appearance, but choosing your doctor is important in order to achieve a natural look.

Ask friends who've already had the injections for recommendations. The manufacturer of Botox has a website listing certified physicians in your area: www.botoxcosmetic.com. You are likely to have the best experience with doctors who are board-certified in dermatology, plastic surgery, or opthalmology or who are ear, nose, and throat specialists.

Who Should Have Botox

Botox is a quick, safe, relatively inexpensive alternative to plastic surgery. "A lot of people say, 'The worry lines on my forehead make me look unhappy and tired,' " Dr. Cook-Bolden says. "Botox is perfect for fading lines that make us appear tired and older."

Botox is a tool that allows you to improve your overall appearance without invasive surgery. The emphasis should be on a natural change. Dr. Cook-Bolden says, "You want to take ethnic differences into consideration. For example, Asian eyes and mouths require special attention. You don't want to overcorrect so that you create an unnatural appearance."

If you're hoping to use Botox instead of undergoing a face-lift, you may be disappointed. Botox won't correct lines that develop as a result of aging, saggy skin. And a smooth brow and eyes free of crow's-feet may actually accentuate sagging skin or puffiness under the eyes. Botox seems to be slightly less effective for people over sixty-five, although Dr. Downie says, "I have a patient who is seventy-four and the Botox injections on her forehead and between her eyes are making a big difference. She looks much more relaxed and younger."

Talk to your physician first to find out what's realistic for you.

The Downside

These injections are a temporary fix. They wear off. That's a good thing if you don't like the results, or if there are side effects. It is possible that your eyelid may droop after the injections, if the substance accidentally migrates into the eyelid muscle. To avoid this, doctors inject you while you are sitting up. It is also important not to bend down for four hours and to avoid exercise the day of the injections. The droopy eyelid syndrome typically lasts about three weeks. Eye drops can help to reverse the problem. But you don't want to have droopy eyelids, and it is a good idea to follow all of the doctor's instructions to prevent causing complications.

COST

Doctors typically set the fees based on the number of areas that are injected. Injections to the forehead area may cost $350 or more. Injections in the forehead and at the bridge of the nose may cost $500. Rates for multiple areas could run as much as $1,500. The cost will vary depending on where you live and the skill of the doctor.

Other Uses

As we mentioned earlier, the botulinum toxin has been used to treat eye muscle and neck and shoulder spasms. Doctors all over the world are now experimenting with a variety of uses. They are injecting the toxin to treat migraines, urinary incontinence, clubfoot in infants, excessive sweating under the arms and on the hands and feet, tennis elbow, carpal tunnel syndrome, jaw pain, vaginal spasms, acid reflux, and even obesity.

The Bottom Line

We like these injections for erasing expression lines safely and temporarily without surgery. But the injections are a medical procedure that requires skill and should be performed by a trained medical professional in a sterile setting. Injection parties are not a good idea.

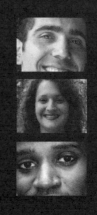

Cancer

CHAPTER 5

THERE'S A SERIOUS AND COMMON MISCONCEPTION THAT PEOPLE with dark skin don't get skin cancer. That is terribly frightening and incorrect. Skin cancer is color-blind and it can be fatal.

In a recent study, Dr. Cook-Bolden and other researchers found that skin cancer is on the rise among African-Americans, Latinos, Asians, and people of Mediterranean, Middle Eastern, and East Indian descent.

In many cases, when it is caught early, a skin cancer, specifically a basal cell cancer, can be treated successfully without a recurrence. Because people with dark and Asian skin assume they're not at risk, however, these cancers frequently aren't detected and can become quite serious. Doctors often make the same erroneous assumption about dark skin, so skin irregularities often aren't caught until it's too late.

Why It Happens

Exposure to the sun's harsh ultraviolet rays is thought to be the number one cause of many skin cancers. The cancerous lesions are most likely to appear on your face, your ears, your neck, and other parts of your body that are exposed to direct sunlight every day.

But the sun isn't the only culprit. It is possible that family history, the cellular makeup of dark and ethnic skin itself, and previous trauma to the skin such as vaccinations, cuts, burns, bruises, radiation, and tattoos may contribute to the development of a skin cancer. At this point, it isn't clear. Research into cancer in dark and ethnic skin has been limited. Until recently it wasn't considered a serious problem. Now, with the number of reported cases of skin cancer rising, more attention is being paid.

Early Warning Signs

Actinic keratosis may be an early warning signal for a squamous cell cancer. These scaly or crusty bumps usually appear on the forehead, ears, cheeks, lips, a bald scalp, the backs of the hands, the forearms, and other areas of the body that have been most frequently exposed to the sun over a period of time.

The appearance of the actinic keratosis may vary slightly depending on its location.

1. Look for red patches on the backs of your hands.
2. Look for scaly patches, or red bumps, on your forehead and scalp.
3. Look for scaly patches, or red or brown patches, on your cheeks and ears.
4. Look for openings filled with dried blood or scaly patches on the lower lip.

These red marks may not be so easy to see in skin of color, and that's why it is important to examine any change in your skin carefully.

Actinic keratosis is often a precancerous lesion. Once the cancer develops, cancerous cells can spread to other parts of the body. A growth found early in its development can often be removed easily or treated in the doctor's office.

"I see these all the time," Dr. Downie says. "Denise, a young woman who'd been a lifeguard all throughout high school and college, came in to my office. She was shocked when I told her that she had an actinic keratosis. She said, 'But my skin is dark. I thought I had protection.' I explained to her that she had spent a good part of her formative years in the sun, and the sun had caused the growth."

Types of Cancer

In skin of color, the common skin cancers include: basal cell carcinoma, squamous cell carcinoma, melanoma, and cutaneous T-cell lymphoma. Although this isn't a medical textbook, we want to arm you with the information you need to spot these cancers before they become more serious. If you know what to look for, you can point it out to your doctor.

Basal Cell Carcinoma

Basal cell carcinoma is the most common type of skin cancer. Although people with fair skin are more likely to develop basal cell carcinoma, olive- and darker-skinned people are not immune.

People who work or play outside in direct sunlight or light reflected from cement, pavement, and water or snow are at the highest risk of developing a basal cell carcinoma. Once upon a time, this cancer was an older person's problem. No more. We see basal cell carcinoma developing in people in their twenties and thirties.

"I recently had a thirty-something African-American patient who lived in the Hamptons on Long Island," Dr. Cook-Bolden says. "He had a medium-brown complexion. He spent a lot of time on the water, and he developed a basal cell cancer on his nose. Fortunately we caught it early. He had surgery, and he now comes back for regular checkups once every three months."

In addition to the sun, there are other risk factors. Basal cell carcinoma is connected frequently to previous traumas: burns, scars, vaccinations, and tattoos. But the sun is usually the most likely cause.

There are five warning signs of a basal cell cancer:

1. A sore that won't heal.
2. A persistent reddish or scaly patch on the arms, chest, legs, or shoulders.
3. A bump that looks pearly or shiny. It can be translucent, pink, red, white, black, or brown.
4. A pink to brown growth that has an indentation in the center and rolled edges. Tiny blood vessels may develop in the center. In darker skin, it might be very dark.
5. A waxy, scarlike area that can be white, yellow, or lighter than normal skin. It is likely to have undefined borders.

TREATMENT

Basal cell carcinomas can be treated and cured. It is possible that after a basal cell carcinoma is removed, it may grow back in the same spot. And unfortunately, if you have a basal cell carcinoma, you are at risk of having more than one. The good news is that this kind of cancer can be treated repeatedly. It won't be life-threatening if you notice the change in your skin at the earliest stages and bring it to the attention of a dermatologist immediately.

Typically your doctor will numb the area with lidocaine and surgically remove the cancer. It is possible that the wound will heal by itself, or the doctor will use stitches to close it.

Many skin cancers are easily shaved off. In this procedure, the doctor removes the affected top layer of skin and stitches aren't necessary.

Large growths may require the skill of a dermatological surgeon.

After the surgeon removes the growth, depending on the location and the size of the wound, the skin is stitched. Although it is possible there will be minimal scarring, the scar size usually reflects the size of the cancer. Your doctor will tell you how to care for the wound at home. It is important to follow the instructions carefully to avoid infection, and to help the wound heal with the faintest scar possible.

TREATMENT OPTIONS

New treatment options also exist that don't require cutting and stitching and therefore leave minimal scarring.

Imiquimod is a topical cream that isn't yet approved by the U.S. Food and Drug Administration for treating cancer. So far it is FDA-approved for treating warts only. Imiquimod stimulates the immune system and triggers the release of chemicals called *cytokines*. Cytokines fight viruses and are thought to destroy cancer cells. Studies are under way to explore Imiquimod's effectiveness in removing small precancerous and cancerous growths.

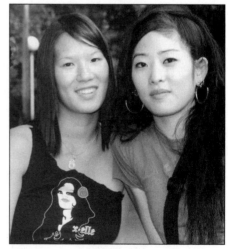

Some researchers are using photodynamic therapy to remove some skin cancers. In this treatment, laser light stimulates a chemical that has been injected into the bloodstream to kill cancerous cells.

When the chemical, called a *photosensitizing agent,* is injected into the bloodstream, it's absorbed by all of the body's cells. The chemical travels through the healthy cells and eventually disappears. But it lingers in the cancerous cells. The doctor then directs a long-wavelength beam of light at the target cells. The photosensitizing agent absorbs the light and a form of oxygen is created that kills the cancerous cells.

The upside of this treatment is that the skin sustains very little 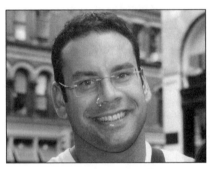 damage. The downside is that you may be uncomfortable for a while. Because the chemical is injected into the bloodstream, it can make your skin and eyes light-sensitive for at least six weeks after the treatment. You'll need to avoid the sun and wear protective clothing if you go outside. Side effects can include coughing, trouble swallowing, stomachaches, and difficulty breathing.

Radiation therapy is another possibility, particularly if a patient is over sixty-five years of age. This treatment is useful if you're fearful of surgery or if you're not healthy enough to endure it. Dr. Downie cautions, "We don't recommend radiation for most people because in some cases, it can cause additional cancerous growths."

Squamous Cell Carcinoma

Squamous cell carcinoma is a very aggressive skin cancer that can spread rapidly. It is often fatal because it isn't detected early enough.

This is one form of skin cancer that people with dark skin can't always blame on the sun. Squamous cell carcinoma can appear on the surface of old injuries, vaccinations, burns, or scars, and even areas on the legs that have been irritated by scratching. It may also appear on the genitals and is often triggered by persistent irritation or trauma caused by sexually transmitted warts or the human papillomavirus.

Recently, Maria asked Dr. Cook-Bolden for help because she had scaly red patches on her right leg. "A biopsy showed that she had squamous cell cancer, and it developed on a spot where Maria had burned her leg when she was a much younger woman," Dr. Cook-Bolden says.

The growth was removed, and Dr. Cook-Bolden is treating Maria with Imiquimod.

WARNING SIGNS

Skin irregularities serve as warning signs.

1. Look for a growth that appears to be a wart. It may crust and bleed.
2. Look for a scaly red patch that won't go away. It isn't well defined and may crust and bleed.
3. Look for a sore that won't heal. It may crust and bleed.
4. Look for a raised mark that grows quickly. It has a dent in the middle and may bleed.
5. Look for a brown or black growth.

TREATMENT

If the growth hasn't spread to muscle or bone, a skilled dermatologist will usually surgically remove it with a scalpel. Frequently these growths dig deep beneath the skin and the dermatologist may have to numb the skin with lidocaine and make a deep incision to remove it. The resulting wound can be stitched in the doctor's office.

More advanced growths require more aggressive treatment. A dermatologic surgeon can perform something called *Mohs micrographic surgery.* This is a highly focused surgery allowing the specialist to remove the cancer without removing a great deal of healthy skin. In this technique, the doctor numbs the skin with a long-acting numbing medication and cuts a thin layer of the skin away. The surgeon then uses a microscope to determine whether any cancer is left. If cancerous cells remain, the same procedure is repeated until all the cells are removed. When the area is clear of cancerous cells, the surgeon will usually repair the wound with stitches.

It is possible that a squamous cell carcinoma that is not caught early may spread to the lymph nodes. If the cancer has spread, your dermatologist will remove the growth and refer you to an oncologist for the appropriate treatment.

A cure is possible. But the cancer must be diagnosed and treated quickly. Sometimes chemotherapy and radiation are necessary.

After a squamous cell carcinoma is removed, a doctor should examine your skin every three to six months for at least the next three years. Dr. Downie says, "We like to encourage patients to be cautious and would prefer that you make this a lifelong practice."

Melanoma

Melanoma tumors begin in the melanocytes—the cells that give your skin color. Melanoma is the most deadly form of skin cancer. If caught early, it can be cured. But too often it is fatal because it spreads beyond the skin to other parts of the body.

Melanoma can occur at any time in your life. Increasingly we see it occurring in people between ages twenty-five and twenty-nine.

Many people don't spot it right away or early enough, because it frequently appears in a preexisting mole. The growth can be tan, brown, black, red, pink, dark blue, or white and is likely to be flat and slightly irregular. This cancer is called *superficial spreading malignant melanoma,* or *SSMM.*

SSMM grows slowly, but once it gets below the superficial layer of skin, it spreads quickly to other parts of the body and is difficult to treat.

Hatira made an appointment with Dr. Cook-Bolden when she noticed that a small, dark mole on her stomach appeared to be growing. Dr. Cook-Bolden did a biopsy.

"It was melanoma and we were lucky to catch it early. The mole was removed before the cancer spread to any other organs or parts of her body," Dr. Cook-Bolden says.

Like other patients who have had a melanoma removed, Hatira now sees Dr. Cook-Bolden for a checkup once every three months.

Acral lentiginous melanoma is the most common form of melanoma in African-Americans, Asians, and Latinos.

It first appears as a black or brown spot under the fingernails or toenails, on the soles of the feet or palms of the hand, or on the genitals. It may look like a bruise or a blood blister, and occasionally it may appear as a blotch. It is dangerous. And it is particularly frightening because this cancer often goes undiagnosed.

"This is a big problem," Dr. Downie says. "When I was in training to be a doctor, a woman named Raquel came in. She'd been bouncing from doctor to doctor. Raquel had a growth underneath her toenail, and doctors kept telling her it was dirt. I discovered that it was an acral lentiginous melanoma. But by the time I found it, the cancer had spread to Raquel's toe, and her toe had to be removed. Raquel is alive and visits a dermatologist for regular checkups once every three months."

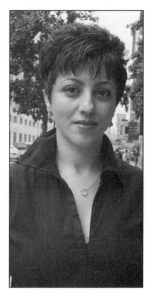

Reggae star Bob Marley wasn't so lucky. He had the same kind of cancer, and it went undiagnosed. He had a small growth underneath a toenail. As it became darker and sore, he dismissed it as a soccer-related bruise. Doctors didn't diagnose it as cancer, and the melanoma spread to his brain and killed him.

Nodular melanoma is the most aggressive form of skin cancer, with a high incidence among Asian people. This skin cancer spreads into deep layers of skin cells much faster than any other type of skin cancer. It usually first appears as a black bump.

Amelanotic melanomas are cancerous growths without pigment. They are typically flesh colored, pinkish, or white growths that suddenly appear and look very different from other moles on your body.

> **IMPORTANT:** *We can't stress how important it is to see a doctor right away, if you have a mark like this that isn't healing.*

Dr. Cook-Bolden says, "The amelanotic melanomas are also very frightening because people often mistake them for pimples, scars, and keloids. We can't stress how important it is to see a doctor right away if you have a mark like this that isn't healing."

WARNING SIGNS

We are going to say it again. Please check your skin regularly. Most of us have blemishes, moles, or freckles. When these change, it may be a sign that something is wrong.

1. Look for changes in size, color, shape, and height.
2. Doctors have developed an ABCD system for spotting atypical moles that may be melanomas:
   A. Asymmetry
   B. Borders that are jagged
   C. Color variation
   D. Diameter over 6 mm, or about one quarter of an inch

TREATMENT

Melanomas that are superficial, aren't too deep in the skin, and are caught early can be removed in the doctor's office. Your dermatologist is likely to numb the area with lidocaine and surgically remove the growth with a scalpel. If the growth is thick or deep, the doctor may have to remove a wider area of the skin. It is possible that the surgeon will perform a skin graft, where healthy skin is taken from another part of your body and is grafted on to the site to repair the damaged skin.

If the melanoma has spread to other parts of your body and surgery is necessary, the dermatologist, depending on his or her training, may perform the operation or recommend the appropriate specialists, including a surgeon and an oncologist.

> **FACT:** *Doctors have developed an ABCD system for spotting atypical moles that may be melanomas:*
>
> **A.** *Asymmetry*
> **B.** *Borders that are jagged*
> **C.** *Color variation*
> **D.** *Diameter over 6 mm, or about one quarter of an inch*

Cutaneous T-Cell Lymphoma

Cutaneous T-cell lymphoma (CTCL), a cancer of the immune system, may begin in the thymus gland or the skin.

CTCL is twice as common in people with dark skin as it is in people with fair skin. And because the cancer can look like eczema or psoriasis, it is another form of cancer that often goes undiagnosed until it has progressed to a dangerous point. Although it is a slow-growing cancer, it can be fatal.

With CTCL you may find patches of scaly skin on your breasts, buttocks, or back. These patches are often confused with other skin problems. If the rash isn't responding to treatment, your doctor should do a thorough examination, consider a skin biopsy, and do blood tests to examine liver function and white and red blood cell count.

WARNING SIGNS

1. You may see red or orange scaly patches.
2. On small patches, your skin may have a cigarette paper look.

3. There may be a mushroomlike growth.

4. You may be losing weight.

5. You may be more tired than usual.

If the skin cancer is caught early, doctors can treat it and prevent it from spreading to other parts of the body. A dermatologist may treat the cancer using a variety of techniques, including application of a topical cream containing mechlorethamine, hydrochloride, or nitrogen mustard. It is possible that the doctor will use a series of ultraviolet light treatments or oral chemotherapeutic agents like Methotrexate.

All treatments depend on the type of cancer and the stage it has reached. If the disease has spread, your dermatologist may recommend a surgeon and an oncologist. It is likely that you'll need chemotherapy, radiation, and other aggressive treatment.

The Bottom Line

These are serious cancers that can kill you. It is important to catch them early. It is doubly important for you to be vigilant because so many doctors assume falsely that skin cancer doesn't strike people with dark skin. Don't hesitate to visit a doctor and ask questions. The questions you ask may save your life.

> IMPORTANT: *Don't hesitate to visit a doctor and ask questions. The questions you ask may save your life.*

Check your skin regularly. At the slightest hint that something is wrong, visit a doctor, preferably a board-certified dermatologist. If the doctor is unfamiliar with something that you are pointing out, ask him or her to look it up, or get a second or third opinion. We know that people are often intimidated when they are in an examining room. But this is no time to be either shy or too polite.

Dr. Downie says, "If you feel you can't afford a visit to your doctor, check with your local hospital. Most offer free skin cancer screening."

Early detection can save your life.

IMPORTANT: *We know that people are often intimidated when they are in an examining room. But this is no time to be either shy or too polite.*

Cellulite

CHAPTER 6

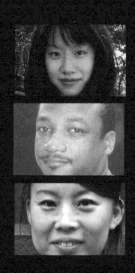

THERE'S NO WAY TO SAY IT SWEETLY. COTTAGE CHEESE THIGHS AND butts aren't pretty.

Unfortunately, 80 percent of all women are thought to have what we've come to call cellulite. Cellulite isn't a medical term. Doctors simply call it fatty tissue. Aestheticians in European spas coined the term and began describing cellulite as a combination of fat, water, and toxic wastes.

"It is a particular problem for African-American, Caribbean-American, and Latina women," Dr. Downie says. "We have to be honest and look at this as an issue that involves your health and your weight. When you think about cellulite, in many cases you have to connect it to the weight problem."

The 2001 United States Surgeon General's report found that obesity is epidemic. The report said that obesity is more common among African-Americans, Caribbean-Americans, Latinos, Native Americans, and Pacific Island Americans than among Asians or Caucasians, but obesity is on the rise in all racial and ethnic groups.

There is a direct correlation between body fat and cellulite. When you gain weight, you are likely to increase your body's cellulite. Many people begin to see cellulite develop right after puberty.

In her e-mail, Dawn describes a classic case of cellulite: "I'm eighteen years old and I'm in desperate need of your help. I'm overweight. I have bad cellulite and I'm embarrassed to wear sleeveless blouses, a bathing suit, or shorts. Is there anything I can do? Will creams work?"

There are things that you can do, but it is unlikely any cream will have a significant effect.

Why It Happens

Cellulite is caused primarily by fat. There's a network of honeycomb chambers made up of muscle and fibers underneath the skin. Your fat is naturally stored in the individual honeycomb compartments. As the fat builds up, the individual chambers fill up and push against the skin. You see the pattern of honeycombs and get the cottage cheesy or waffly look because the chambers are bulging.

Women are more likely than men to see cellulite because men have thicker skin, and their fat storage compartments have a different structural pattern. Estrogen also plays a role. The higher your estrogen level, the more likely you are to have cellulite. Consequently, some men, and even thin women, may develop cellulite. Researchers also think family history may determine whether we form cellulite.

Remedies
What You Can Do on Your Own

You may need to revolutionize your diet and your lifestyle. Your skin is the beautiful wrapping for your total package, and it reflects everything that you put into your body. The more fat you take in, the more likely you are to see the bulges of cellulite.

There's no quick or easy solution. This is another area in which the improved management of your daily routine can significantly improve your overall health and the beauty of your skin.

A balanced diet and regular exercise program will go a long way toward reducing fat and eliminating most of the cellulite.

DIET

You don't have to have a complicated diet program. But you do need to reduce the amount of sugar you eat and drink. You want to avoid fatty foods and fried foods. For a healthy diet, eat fish, lean meat, fruits, vegetables, and whole grains. Instead of sugary drinks, try water. We recommend eight to ten glasses a day. The water keeps tissues healthy by moving everything through the body.

IMPORTANT: *You may need to revolutionize your diet and your lifestyle. Your skin is the beautiful wrapping for your total package, and it reflects everything that you put into your body.*

EXERCISE

A regular cardiovascular exercise program that burns fat and calories is also important. Whether you choose to jog on the street, run or walk on the treadmill at a gym, or swim in a pool, cardiovascular exercise for at least thirty minutes a session three times a week is essential. Dr. Downie says, "It's much better to try to control cellulite with exercise rather than liposuction or another expensive fat reduction technique."

In addition, a weight workout will help you tone your muscles. Don't worry about building bulging muscles. It is difficult for women to bulk up. Unless you're a body builder on steroids, you won't develop a masculine-looking body.

Free weights of more than ten pounds and gym equipment that provides resistance can help to reshape your body and reduce the cellulite. It is a good idea to work with someone in the gym at least once to become familiar with the equipment and to make sure that you are using it safely. Use the maximum amount of weight you are comfortable with and build on that. Push yourself—but do it carefully.

David Fitzpatrick, a trainer at Crunch gyms, says, "Don't reach for the lightest weight; you'll be wasting your time. Very heavy weights are good, but if you are not careful you may hurt yourself. If you are working out alone, I recommend using medium weights." Fitzpatrick suggests testing the weights to see how much weight you can move up and down repeatedly.

To burn fat and build muscle, he recommends that you establish a routine and do a variety of weight exercises in series of twelve to fifteen repetitions. Fitzpatrick also advises, "If you are working out alone, the weight machines are generally safer because they target specific muscles and it is more difficult to do the exercises incorrectly."

Yoga workouts in which exercises are performed repeatedly and consistently also condition the body and can help to decrease cellulite over time.

Moisturize

There is one more step to take; moisturizing the skin while you are dieting and exercising can help to improve your skin's elasticity. Cetaphil, Lubriderm, Eucerin, and Curel are good all-purpose moisturizers. Vanicream and SBR Lipocream are thick moisturizers that are particularly good for dry skin.

A Doctor's Guidance

Before you begin an exercise program, check with your physician to make sure that you are healthy and can fully participate in all activities.

If you are overweight or obese, it is essential that you see a doctor to develop a weight loss and exercise plan that is realistic. Once you begin to lose weight and tone your muscles, you'll feel better and have more energy. There is bound to be a reduction in the amount of cellulite. If the cellulite is persistent, you may want to talk with a board-certified dermatologist or plastic surgeon about liposuction.

Liposuction

Although we generally like liposuction—the vacuuming method that removes fat from under the skin—it isn't always effective for reducing cellulite. Liposuction removes fat and reduces fat cells in a specific place. But if you continue to ingest fat and build it up in your body, the new fat will migrate to another portion of the body that was untouched by liposuction. With new fat in new places, you may end up with more cellulite than you had to begin with.

It is important that you communicate with your doctor. Explain what you expect. And listen to the doctor's explanation. You may not be able to achieve your dream reduction. Even if liposuction worked for your girlfriends, it may not erase your cellulite. And who wants to waste money on a procedure that doesn't give you the best results? We'll talk more about liposuction in chapter 25.

Creams and Dreams

Snake oil salespeople are promoting thigh-reducing creams, herbal remedies, and special pills on television, on the Internet, and over the telephone. It's a billion-dollar business that makes some people rich, but it may leave you a little poorer and still stuck with the same old cellulite.

Many of these products contain a combination of herbs, oils, and caffeine. They promise to attack the cellulite by reducing fluid buildup, knocking out fat at the source, increasing blood circulation, and stimulating metabolism. The U.S. Food and Drug Administration has cited many companies for making false and misleading claims, but the false practices continue. Be aware that some companies take advantage of your eagerness for quick results. None of these products has been scientifically proven effective to eliminate cellulite.

Rolling the Fat Away

Some companies claim that their machines roll and suck, or squeeze, the cellulite away. A process called Endermologie, created in France, has been approved by the FDA for temporarily reducing the appearance of cellulite. It is a nonsurgical method performed with a hand-held, motorized device that rolls, folds, and suctions the surface of the skin. The process theoretically breaks up fat and stimulates blood flow.

People who have had at least twenty sessions do see some improvement. But when they stop the treatments, their cellulite comes right back. Even the believers say it must be combined with a weight loss and exercise program. For it to be effective, it requires a serious commitment of time and money. We're not fans of this process, but some people like it. "You must be realistic and understand that it is not a miracle cure. It doesn't work for everyone and it won't work without diet and exercise," says Dr. Cook-Bolden.

Combination Therapies

Some doctors are combining Endermologie with light or laser therapies. They theorize that light and laser systems heat up the fat and make it easier to massage during the Endermologie process. But this combination treatment hasn't been widely researched. Dr. Downie says, "I'm concerned about using light and laser therapy in this way. It could lead to burns and severe scarring or keloids. People with skin of color must be very careful."

The Bottom Line

We won't list every so-called miracle cure that is on the market today. But the simple facts of anatomy and body chemistry tell us that there is no substitute for a healthy diet and a good exercise routine. You may never be completely cellulite-free. But you can reduce the amount of fat in your body and consequently the pattern the fat makes on your skin.

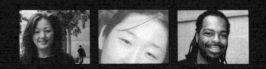

Chemical
Peels

CHAPTER 7

CLEOPATRA UNDERSTOOD THE CURRENCY OF GOOD LOOKS AND enhanced her power by using the mystique of beauty. We're told that Cleopatra regularly luxuriated in milk baths to make her skin smooth, soft, and supple. Although she's the most celebrated historical figure who reportedly bathed in milk or lactic acid to exfoliate the top layers of dead skin, we're not sure when the practice started. Asians, Egyptians, the Greeks, and the Romans all knew the secret of natural chemical peels and their ability to rejuvenate the skin. Even in the Middle Ages, rich Europeans improved the texture of their skin and their overall appearance by applying the tartaric acid from aged wine.

Today we use natural and synthetic chemical peels to renew our skin, fade fine lines around the eyes and mouth, even out skin tone, and treat acne. But if you have Asian, olive, or dark skin, you may be wondering about safety. Vita writes, "I'm of East Indian descent and I have a lot of dark spots. Will chemical peels help, or will they harm my dark skin?"

It was the dark-skinned people of the hills and valleys of Asia and India, the countries surrounding the Mediterranean, and the deserts of the Middle East who first discovered the healing properties of natural acids.

People with skin of color can be treated with chemical peels safely, but when used incorrectly, the same peels may cause much damage.

"Everyone with skin of color must be careful that they have the right strength and type of peel for their skin," Dr. Cook-Bolden cautions. "It is particularly important to remember that Asian skin is easily damaged. We think that's because the melanocytes, the pigment-producing cells, can react much more unpredictably in Asian skin than the melanocytes in other ethnic skin."

But when properly and safely used, chemical peels are useful on all areas of the body. They can even out skin tone, erase discoloration, and make the skin look healthier and younger. "Chemical peels are one of the most popular cosmetic procedures. We use chemical peels all the time to help people fade the fine lines on their faces. We also use peels regularly to help control acne," Dr. Cook-Bolden says.

How It Works

Our skin is constantly renewing itself. Surface skin cells continuously wear away and are immediately replaced by another set of cells. Every four to five weeks we have a new outer layer of skin that can be healthier and fresher looking. By using a chemical peel, we take control of the renewal process and speed it up.

"Chemical peels are an important part of a management plan for healthy, attractive skin," Dr. Downie says. "I give myself a chemical peel once a month. It helps me maintain an even skin tone and decreases the acne that flares up from time to time."

Our methodology may be more sophisticated now, but the ingredients in our chemical peels are very similar to those in the preparations Cleopatra used.

Natural alpha and beta hydroxy acids are derived from plants, fruits, and milk. Glycolic acid, which is in many cosmetic preparations, was originally made from sugarcane. Beta hydroxy acid in its natural form is found in the bark of the white willow tree and the wintergreen plant.

Beta hydroxy acid, or salicylic acid, is especially good for people with oily skin, and for inflammatory conditions like acne and rosacea.

Since it's not practical to extract these acids for a mass market, scientists created synthetic copies. Both the natural acids and the synthetics work the same way. They speed up the skin's natural renewal cycle.

Chemical peels loosen the bonds that hold the old cells together. They also stimulate the body's natural collagen. This is very beneficial because collagen is the fibrous protein that makes our skin smooth and plumps it up. When collagen wears down, the skin sags, and fine lines develop. Collagen renewal helps to tone the skin and fill in the fine lines.

Chemical peels and retinoids, which are derivatives of vitamin A, work on the same principle. Retinoids also stimulate collagen and renew the skin. But they must be used regularly over a long period of time to be effective. Many people incorporate a retinoid into a regular nightly routine that they maintain for years to create healthier, smoother skin. Retinoids are used in topical creams like Renova, Retin-A Micro, Differin, and Avage. Typically, you apply a pea-size amount to your face nightly or several times a week. Dermatologists often prescribe retinoids for your at-home regimen to complement a series of chemical peels. We've found that many therapies work better together. Chemical peels and retinoids are an excellent example; one enhances the effectiveness of the other.

When a chemical peel is applied, the amount of acid in the peels may vary from 20 percent to 99 percent of acid in the solution. Most dermatologists begin with a 20 to 35 percent solution. And if the patient can tolerate it, the doctor moves toward the 70 percent range and sometimes to 99 percent. The higher the acidic content in the solution, the stronger the peel and the more irritated the skin gets. This is an important consideration for people with skin of color.

The melanocytes that give the skin pigment are normally very active in skin of color. It is easy to overstimulate them and create dark marks and blotches. A peel administered by the wrong hands, and particularly one that is too strong, can easily do damage.

Milder, or superficial, peels are often called "lunchtime peels." They may make your skin a bit red for a short time, but you should be able to go back to work or out immediately following the peel.

Medium-depth peels, with a solution of trichloracetic acid, or TCA, are not for everyone because of their intensity.

Roxanne was fifty-two years old when the discoloration on her face began to bother her. She went to see Dr. Cook-Bolden, who recommended a series of trichloracetic acid peels. "She had medium- to light-dark skin," Dr. Cook-Bolden says. "I used a thirty-five percent solution of trichloracetic acid in a peel. It worked so well to remove the splotchiness that we only had to do two peels."

This is *not* a lunchtime peel. It does require healing time.

We want to warn you that the TCA peel can be uncomfortable, and it may take ten to twelve days for the skin to lose the redness and barklike flakiness as the skin sloughs off. It is imperative to repeatedly apply a healthy dose of oil-free moisturizer to the skin until the new skin cells settle in. It is also essential to wear sun protection during the time you are having the peels and long after.

Dermatologists who regularly administer chemical peels are likely to mix custom-made solutions. They can gauge what works best for your skin and create an individual program.

A Doctor's Guidance

We can't say it frequently enough: Skin sensitivity varies, and it is important to find a doctor who understands skin of color and the need to treat it gently.

You may not get instant results, but if you are consistent and willing to have regular peels, there can be a dramatic improvement.

Carol visited Dr. Downie's office a year and a half before her wedding. At twenty-nine, she still had the acne that had plagued her since her teen years. She had acne bumps and an uneven skin tone. Carol camouflaged her problem with heavy makeup; in fact, her fiancé had never seen her without it. But she didn't want to hide behind a veil of cosmetics forever.

Dr. Downie administered a series of strong glycolic acid peels; she began with a 70 percent solution and gradually increased the strength. After four treatments, Dr. Downie switched to more potent salicylic acid peels and continued these peels once a month for a little over a year. "The results were amazing. It decreased the amount of acne breakouts, smoothed the texture of Carol's skin, and evened out her skin tone," Dr. Downie says.

Carol wore very little makeup on her wedding day, and now Carol has a salicylic chemical peel once every three months.

The moral of this story is that planning and management are required if you want to have beautiful skin for a special day. Carol's story also illustrates the importance of continuing a program that you've devised with a doctor you trust.

Very strong peels, or deep peels like phenol peels, are too strong for skin of color. We don't recommend them. It is common to see blistering, redness, and irritation for weeks and perhaps months. When the irritation subsides, people with skin of color are likely to develop dark spots or light blotches as a direct result of the strong peel.

If you are using a retinoid like Retin-A Micro, Renova, Differin, Avage, or Tazorac, it is a good idea to stop five to seven days before the peel. You don't want your skin to be supersensitive when the peel is applied.

Who Administers the Peel

Chemical peels are very popular, and aestheticians often apply peels as part of a facial routine. In many states aestheticians are allowed to administer only the most superficial peels. Dermatologists and plastic surgeons regularly use chemical peels of all strengths. But whoever applies the peel must understand how to treat dark skin.

What to Expect

We like to apply the peel on the face and down the neck, and sometimes over the collar bone just above the chest if it is necessary. The areas should be cleansed and makeup free. The solution will be swabbed on quickly. Everyone has a different tolerance level. It is important to communicate with the person applying the peel if you experience discomfort.

We ask patients to tell us on a scale of one to ten how much burning or tingling they feel. Don't be a martyr. We'll stop before you get to ten. The solution will sting, and it's likely to remain on your face for five minutes or less. The time will vary depending on the strength of the solution, the area being treated, and your tolerance. On some areas of the body the solution may stay on for a longer period of time. When the time is up, there's a thorough rinse with cool water or another type of neutralizer.

We administer the peels in a series of six to twelve sessions given once every two to four weeks. By spreading out the peels, we get the results we want without irritating the skin too much.

COST

Chemical peels vary in price. They are likely to range from $250 to $2,000, depending on the area being treated and the type of peel.

The Bottom Line

Chemical peels are a useful tool in an overall skin management routine. Finding the right doctor is important. Get recommendations from friends who've already had a series of successful peels. The websites of the American Academy of Dermatology and the American Society for Dermatologic Surgery are good tools for finding a qualified dermatologist in your area. You can reach them at www.aad.org, and www.aboutskinsurgery.com.

To get the most benefit from the peels, it will be necessary to follow through on all of the doctor's recommendations.

After a peel, sunblock is a must. Your skin will be sensitive, and the sun can too easily stimulate the pigment cells, which will create dark spots. Protect yourself and your investment in your skin by wearing sun protection with Parsol 1789, UVA and UVB protection, and a sun protection factor of between 20 and 30, with zinc oxide or titanium dioxide. Always remember to apply it every two hours.

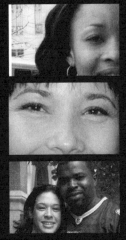

Collagen and Wrinkle Fillers

CHAPTER 8

COLLAGEN INJECTIONS AND WRINKLE FILLERS ARE PURELY COSMETIC procedures that are really all about you. Currently, injectable collagen is the most widely used wrinkle filler; it is a quick, relatively inexpensive, and almost painless way to improve your appearance.

Jean e-mailed: "I have deep furrows alongside my mouth. Will collagen work? Is it okay for dark skin?"

We'll start backward. Collagen is perfectly safe for dark skin. And it is perfect for the deep lines that run down from your nose to your mouth and make you look older than you feel.

"I love doing collagen," Dr. Downie says. "People are very excited to see instant results. And as I inject someone, she or he can look in the mirror and watch the change take place."

How Collagen Works

All of us naturally have collagen in our bodies. This strong, fibrous protein is a central part of our body's architecture. Collagen helps to hold everything together. It is in our bones, muscles, joints, tendons, blood vessels, and many organs, including the skin, where it plays an extremely important role. Seventy-five percent of the skin is collagen. It provides a lattice or meshlike underpinning to hold and support the skin cells. Collagen gives the skin resilience, shape, and texture. Because of collagen we have the full, soft, unlined look we take for granted when we are young. And what nature giveth, nature taketh away.

Collagen wears out. Years of smiling, frowning, squinting, and assorted facial expressions wear the natural collagen down. We see the results most obviously with lines and wrinkles. There's simply not enough collagen left in the skin to plump it up and fill out the lines.

Collagen works from the inside out. You can't slather it on your skin and expect it to work. Those highly touted collagen creams don't get below the surface of the skin. As we describe in other chapters, retinoid creams used over time, alpha and beta hydroxy products and peels, some vitamin therapies, laser treatments, and other new innovations that penetrate the skin and stimulate the collagen can cause what doctors call "collagen remodeling."

But if you are looking for instant results in specific areas, collagen injections are an effective way to go. When collagen is injected, it becomes a filler underneath the lines and wrinkles, plumping them up like your natural collagen once did.

Collagen is used to fill in the deep lines on either side of your mouth. These so-called puppet lines are filled easily with collagen. Forehead and frown lines can also be filled in with collagen. We inject collagen to fill in acne scars, smile lines, and tiny vertical lip lines, as well as crow's-feet. We also like to use it to plump up the skin of the hands, giving them a more youthful appearance. And increasingly, collagen is being used in conjunction with Botox to rejuvenate aging faces and necks.

You've seen pictures of people with lips suddenly puffed by collagen. It doesn't have to be that way. Collagen, when used correctly, can improve the natural contour of the lips.

Sonia wrote asking for advice: "I'm a forty-something African-American woman. Don't laugh. My lips aren't full. They are getting thinner as I get older. Now it looks like I don't have an upper lip. Can I do anything about this without having surgery?"

Collagen is a possible answer. "The way the collagen is injected must be controlled," Dr. Downie warns. "Many people overdo it. And that's why you have the infamous cases of pillow lips."

If administered properly, collagen can achieve an almost natural look, and it won't interfere with kissing, eating, or any other important functions.

Where Collagen Comes From

The most widely used collagen is extracted from cows and purified, refined, and manufactured into an injectable substance. In the 1970s doctors and researchers discovered that cow collagen was so close to human collagen that it could be used effectively to help repair damaged skin.

INAMED Aesthetics, the company that harvests and manufactures bovine collagen approved for use in the United States, says it uses collagen only from a select herd of cows. And it oversees the breeding of this "closed herd" to ensure that none of the cows used for harvesting are contaminated by other cows or by what they eat. Until recently this has been the primary source of injectable collagen used by doctors. But now INAMED has produced another type of collagen that may prove easier and quicker to use. The company has created a human collagen purified from skin tissue and grown in controlled laboratory conditions. The FDA has approved this type of human collagen as injectable fillers.

A Doctor's Guidance

Before a series of shots begins, a doctor will test you to see if you are allergic to the collagen. A small amount of collagen will be injected into your forearm. INAMED recommends that a patient wait four weeks to make sure there's no redness, itching, or swelling. Then, INAMED suggests testing again and waiting another four weeks. Many doctors and patients don't wait the full four or eight weeks. They do the testing in two-week intervals because they are eager to complete the test injections. Some settle for one test. In most cases, the cow collagen is administered without any problems.

The newer human-based collagen has an advantage. It doesn't require testing and can be administered the same day you visit a doctor.

How Collagen Is Administered

Collagen is premixed with the anesthetic lidocaine. Unless you're supersensitive, you won't need anything else to numb the area. Some doctors may apply a numbing cream. "I'm not in favor of that technique," Dr. Cook-Bolden says. "Anesthetics can blur the natural contour of the face and I prefer to inject the collagen without numbing."

The manufacturer has created two types of cow and human collagen. Zyderm, a cow collagen, and CosmoDerm, collagen bioengineered from human collagen, are used to treat superficial wrinkles, lines, and scars. Zyplast (cow) and CosmoPlast (human) are used for the deeper lines and wrinkles. It is a good idea to let your doctor decide which one you need.

Regardless of the type of collagen, the doctor will use a fine needle and inject the substance at several points along the line or scar. In some cases, the doctor may inject more collagen on one side of the face to help match the natural symmetry. It may seem a little lopsided until the collagen settles. When the injections are completed, you may have some redness or swelling. Both usually disappear within a few days. Because the collagen is in a saline solution, the injected area may initially look like it is very puffy until your body absorbs the saline. That may take a few hours, or a day or two.

"Collagen is a wonderful way to fill in facial lines," Dr. Cook-Bolden says. But she warns, "With skin of color you want to make sure that you inject the collagen very gingerly. You don't want to traumatize the skin and provoke the cells to produce more color. If the doctor isn't careful, you can get dark marks at the site of the injections."

Temporary Results

The results from collagen injections are only temporary. They may last between three and six months depending on how your body absorbs the collagen. Studies have found that in some people, collagen injections stimulate natural collagen, prolonging the effect.

The Downside

Again, there is the possibility of an allergic reaction, which is why it is important to test first. Some people can see the collagen implant under the skin as a fine bump, white spots, or red, hivelike bumps. There also have been reports of people who have developed connective tissue disease after collagen injections. But it is important to note that there have been conflicting studies about collagen and long-term problems.

Dr. Downie says, "The new human-based collagen may be better for allergy-prone people and those who couldn't have collagen injections in the past."

COST

Doctors generally charge you for the amount of collagen that is injected. The cost could range from $350 to $1,000. It will vary depending on the skill of the doctor and where you live.

Wrinkle Fillers

Although collagen is the most widely used wrinkle filler, many doctors are using other substances and methods. Some are being used in

Europe and elsewhere but are not yet approved in the United States. Researchers are performing clinical trials on these products in the hope that they will be able to market them in the United States.

Artecoll

Some doctors are using Artecoll, an injectable substance made of tiny plastic beads suspended in cow collagen mixed with lidocaine and a saline solution. Artecoll is considered a permanent filler. Doctors inject Artecoll the same way they inject collagen. After the injections, there may be some redness or swelling for a week.

The filler becomes permanent as the body's natural collagen wraps around the tiny plastic beads. This process takes about three months. At this point, the cow collagen will have dissolved, and your doctor may recommend a second set of injections to fill the wrinkles more fully. Initial studies in the United States recommend it for facial wrinkles except for around the mouth; doctors found that in some people it caused tiny bumps in the skin in the mouth area. Artecoll is used in Europe and elsewhere and is under consideration for approval by the U.S. Food and Drug Administration.

COST

Doctors injecting Artecoll typically charge $400 to $900 per injection, depending on the number of injections and the areas being treated.

Calcium Hydroxyapatite

Calcium hydroxyapatite is a mineral that we all have in our bones and teeth. Doctors have been using versions of calcium hydroxyapatite for chin and other facial implants for many years. Now BioForm has created a synthetic, injectable form of calcium hydroxyapatite and is marketing it under the name Radiance. Although the FDA hasn't approved Radiance as a wrinkle filler, it is approved for other uses. Radiance is widely used in Europe for filling lines and wrinkles, and a growing number of doctors in the United States are also using it as a wrinkle filler because it is relatively long-lasting.

Some doctors find Radiance particularly effective for filling in the lines that run between the nose and mouth, the furrows over the bridge of the nose, and the deep hollows that appear in the cheeks as a result of AIDS-related illnesses. On the downside, doctors have discovered that tiny bumps may appear after Radiance is injected into the lip area, so they suggest that it not be used there.

Radiance does not require a skin test. It is injected in the doctor's office without a numbing agent. Icing the area immediately after the injection should decrease any redness or swelling that might occur. Redness and swelling should disappear within twenty-four hours.

Over time, natural collagen develops around the Radiance to hold it in place for two years or more.

COST

The cost of the injections can range from $400 to $1,500 depending on the area being treated.

Fat Transplantation

Doctors have harvested fat to fill scars for more than a hundred years. Some doctors now use your body's fat to fill facial wrinkles and plump up lips and hands. The procedure is relatively simple. Fat is usually removed from your thighs, buttocks, tummy, or knees. To remove the fat, the doctor will treat the area with a local anesthetic and draw out the fat with a long needle attached to a suction device. The fat is then purified: the fat cells are separated from the blood cells and prepared for the transfer. A long needle is used to insert the fat into the target area. Some puffiness or swelling may occur until the fat is absorbed. And there may be some bruising or redness for a few days. In some people the fat transfer can last a year or more, but others have seen the fat dissolve within a month.

COST
Fat injections are likely to cost $1,000 and up depending on the area being treated.

Hyaluronic Acid
Hyaluronic acid is a jellylike substance that is naturally found in our bodies. It helps the skin retain water, cushions and lubricates the skin, and also helps deliver important nutrients from the bloodstream to skin cells. Like collagen, it wears out. Researchers have developed injectable synthetic forms of hyaluronic acid to plump up the skin and fill in moderate lines and wrinkles. Companies are marketing them under the brand names Restylane, Hylaform, and Perlane. The FDA has approved Restylane.

It's injected, like collagen, with a fine needle. Some swelling or redness may occur at the site of the injection that could last for a week. Dr. Downie says, "Restylane doesn't require a skin test. There's no waiting period, and it may last six months or longer."

COST
Restylane injections are likely to cost between $400 and $1,500 depending on the areas being injected.

Sculptra
Manufactured by Dermik Laboratories, Sculptra is a biodegradable, injectable poly-L-lactic acid that fills deep lines, wrinkles, and scars. It is FDA approved for use in HIV patients with facial fat loss, but

because it also thickens the skin by stimulating your natural collagen, many doctors are using Sculptra as a filler for various cosmetic patients. A skin test isn't required before an injection, but you may experience bruising, swelling, or the formation of small bumps around the area of the injection. The bruising and swelling should disappear in a few days, but the small bumps may remain for several months. You may need more than one session to fill deep lines or scars.

COST
Sculptra injections are likely to cost $1,000 to $1,500 depending upon the areas being treated.

Silicone
Silicone implants for wrinkles are illegal in the United States. Some doctors and aestheticians are misusing these implants. We have seen bumps, permanent swelling, and unsightly bulges from scar tissue formations that develop years after the silicone has been injected.

Some dermatologists and researchers are, however, conducting tests with liquid, medical-grade injectable silicone to see if it can be used safely and effectively.

The Bottom Line
Choose your doctor carefully. The effectiveness and safety of wrinkle fillers depend on the skill of the doctor performing the procedure. Ask your friends for recommendations or visit the websites of the American Academy of Dermatology and the American Society for Dermatologic Surgery to find qualified doctors in your area. The website addresses are www.aad.org and www.aboutskinsurgery.org.

Cysts ——

CHAPTER 9

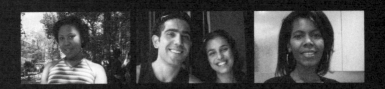

MOST NONACNE CYSTS MATERIALIZE OUT OF THE BLUE AND CAN BE very painful and very frustrating.

Daphne asks the questions we hear all the time: "I get these painful lumps on my scalp and forehead. Is there anything I can do to prevent them and get rid of them permanently?"

We wish we had different answers. Cysts can't be prevented. When they appear, they should be treated. Some cysts can be removed, but they may grow back either in the same place or in a new spot.

Why It Happens

Researchers really don't know why a nonacne cyst develops. There are only theories to explain the occurrence of nonacne cysts, from clogged pores to hereditary causes to the possibility that they exist under the skin from the time we're born and get larger and push out to the skin's surface as we get older.

Cysts appear as bumps on the scalp, face, neck, back, underarms, buttocks, and in the groin and on the scrotum, where they can be very painful.

Cysts usually aren't cancerous, but they should be checked by a doctor. A foul odor is a warning sign that you need medical treatment. Cysts often get inflamed, fill with pus, and can become infected. It is important to get treatment quickly.

Remedies

What You Can Do on Your Own

If the cyst is small and doesn't trouble you, it is often best to leave it alone. When a cyst is inflamed or has a black dot in the center, you may be tempted to squeeze it. Don't do it! You'll be on the road to infection and possible scarring.

Instead, wet a clean washcloth with warm water, and gently place this soothing compress over it. We also find that swabbing the cyst with benzoyl peroxide is another good way to ease the inflammation and the pain.

A Doctor's Guidance

You may need a doctor's help. Dr. Downie says, "Mark came into my office with several cysts. He had a terrible infection because he hadn't taken proper care of them. I had to admit him to the hospital so that he could receive intravenous antibiotics."

The possibility of infection is a particular problem for people who suffer from diabetes because they are more susceptible to superficial bacterial infections.

If the cyst is filled with fluid, the doctor will likely make a small opening to drain it. When a cyst is painful, a doctor may inject it with a mild cortisone. In some cases the doctor will numb the area and remove it surgically. Cysts, unfortunately, may grow back and have to be removed again.

Prescription Medicines

In addition to cortisone and antibiotic creams, a doctor may prescribe oral antibiotics like Keflex, or anti-inflammatories like prednisone for a limited time in very severe cases. People who have persistently painful cysts may require a tetracycline like Dynacin or Doryx for at least six months. In extreme cases, a doctor might prescribe Accutane, the antiacne medication, which helps to stop the oil production and the development of the cysts. But there are strict guidelines for pre-scribing and taking Accutane or generic versions of the drug. It requires blood tests and close monitoring because there are serious potential side effects, described in the acne chapter (see pages 30–31).

The Bottom Line

A cyst should not be ignored. Have it treated by a doctor. Because Asian, olive, and dark skin is easily marred, a cyst that becomes inflamed or infected can easily leave a dark mark. That's why it is also important to seek out a doctor who understands skin of color and who will treat you in a way that won't damage your skin.

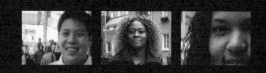

Dangerous
Products

CHAPTER 10

CONSIDER THIS A SERIOUS WARNING: A FADE CREAM OR SOAP THAT you've been using to lighten dark spots, or to even out your skin tone, may be hurting you. You may not notice anything immediately. Your problem may even improve for a while. Over time the cosmetic problem that you thought you were solving will suddenly look worse.

> **IMPORTANT:** *Consider this a serious warning: a fade cream or soap that you've been using to lighten dark spots, or to even out your skin tone, may be hurting you.*

Many of these products are popular. They are sold in neighborhood stores and are available over the Internet. But they can be dangerous enough to hurt you and your children.

We have found these illegally imported products, aimed at lightening Asian, olive, and dark skin, in a wide variety of stores in many ethnic neighborhoods. Although they are touted as miracle creams, they can be extremely damaging, with long-term cosmetic and health consequences.

Some people find out about the side effects only after the damage is done. Riccardo wrote to us about his mistake: "I have burns from a bleaching cream that I bought in my neighborhood store. I tried it to lighten dark spots on my face. My skin burned and now it is even blotchier." Diana had a similar experience: "I'm a Caribbean-American and my friends recommended a cream to fade the dark spots on my face. Now I have lighter marks and you can see tiny red veins."

Riccardo and Diana used creams to fade dark marks. But many people buy these creams and soaps in a futile and dangerous attempt to change their skin color.

Danny is a teenager who asked us for a recommendation that we wouldn't dream of making even if we could: "I'm West Indian. People always mistake me for being African. What can I do to get rid of my dark skin?" We received the same request from Sita in an e-mail: "We are Indian and my daughter has darker skin than the rest of the family. Is there anything that I can do to make it lighter?"

Please do nothing. Look in the mirror and love yourself for who you are. Dark skin is beautiful. There is no reason on earth to lighten it.

We know that thousands of people like Danny and Sita all over the world are attempting to lighten their skin and their children's skin with dangerous products. Millions of others like Riccardo and Diana try to correct a cosmetic problem and make it worse by using a dangerous product. Dr. Downie says, "In addition to causing health problems, skin lighteners also create uneven skin tones. They can also make the skin an unnatural color. This damage is very difficult to reverse. A number of celebrities have come to me recently after using these products, and they are struggling with the consequences of serious damage."

> **OUR THOUGHTS:** *Look in the mirror and love yourself for who you are. Dark skin is beautiful. There is no reason on earth to lighten it.*

We will talk about safe ways to treat dark spots and uneven skin tone in chapter 12 (see pages 121–125). But in this chapter we want to provide the information you need about unsafe products.

Beware

Beware of over-the-counter creams, gels, and soaps containing mercury, steroids, and prescription-strength hydroquinone. These products are not approved for sale over the counter in the United States.

Products containing mercury are banned by the European Union, although many are manufactured in Europe and exported to Africa, Asia, Latin America, and the Caribbean and then make their way into the United States.

Initially the products seem to work, which is why they became popular. People talk about the "miraculous changes." The word gets passed along a poisonous grapevine. When the problems begin, the talking stops. It is often too embarrassing to admit that you've made a mistake and hurt yourself.

Mercury

The mercury in these soaps, creams, ointments, and gels is enough to cause enormous concern. The popular products Movate Germicidal Soap and Roberts Medicated Soap are two that we have purchased, in neighborhood stores, as part of our investigation. Both contain mercury, and the ingredient is listed clearly on their labels.

Using these soaps, or any other mercury-based product or cream, is dangerous. Many people who use the mercury-based products compound its harmful effects by lathering the soap or cream on the skin, allowing it to dry overnight, and washing it off the next morning. This is terribly dangerous.

Over time, mercury can damage the skin, leaving patches that are rough and black, green, or red. It is also possible to develop skin cancer as a result of prolonged use of mercury-based products. Mercury poisoning can cause brain damage and kidney failure. Once the mercury enters the bloodstream, it is difficult to eliminate.

The World Health Organization found that when mercury enters a mother's system, she can pass it on to her unborn child.

Dr. Cook-Bolden says, "Women come in after using these mercury-based products complaining they have no feeling in their legs or arms. It's a bad sign that they have nerve damage caused by mercury poisoning."

Hydroquinone

Hydroquinone is used effectively by dermatologists to fade dark spots and even out skin tone because it blocks the production of the enzyme tyrosinase in the melanocyte cells that give the skin color. Products like Alustra, Lustra-AF, Glyquin XM, Tri-Luma Cream, and EpiQuin Micro containing 4 percent hydroquinone are prescribed by doctors, who sometimes also prescribe products with higher strengths of hydroquinone to treat medical and cosmetic conditions.

In the United States, the Food and Drug Administration allows you to buy over-the-counter products that contain 2 percent hydro-

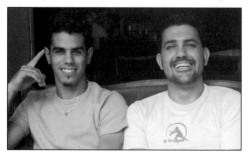

quinone. But we have found dangerous products on store shelves containing more than the legal amount.

People who use prescription-strength hydroquinone without a doctor's supervision run the risk of developing a blotchy, severely uneven skin tone that may be impossible to correct.

Hydroquinone is tightly regulated and even banned in parts of Europe and throughout Asia. Studies have shown that high concentrations and prolonged use may cause cancer and other side effects, including permanent white patches and irritation. There have also been reports that in rare cases hydroquinone caused thick raised scars called keloids.

Cortisone

Cortisone, also regulated by the U.S. Food and Drug Administration, is a steroid that doctors use to treat inflammation. Milder forms are available over the counter legally. But stronger forms used over a prolonged period of time can thin the skin.

Although people buy these products to use on their faces, doctors rarely prescribe very strong cortisone for the face because they don't want to damage the skin. When it is prescribed, we usually ask you to use it for only two weeks under a doctor's careful supervision. These steroids lighten the skin as a side effect, and doctors use them in a controlled way.

When you apply these products on your own, without a prescription and without a doctor's guidance, you're likely to use too much. You can easily thin the skin on your face, create permanent white depigmented blotches, and develop tiny red capillaries and other marks that are difficult to treat.

Many of these dangerous products contain the steroid betamethasone. If you use it for too long, it can weaken your immune system. It is very dangerous for people who have serious health problems, including diabetes and other endocrine diseases.

Pregnant women run the risk of hurting their unborn babies. Doctors limit the use of all medications, including betamethasone, during pregnancy unless absolutely necessary. And the research isn't yet conclusive about the effects of betamethasone on pregnant women. We do know that mothers can pass betamethasone on to their infants through breast milk, creating a potentially dangerous situation for the babies.

Other creams include the stronger steroid clobetasol propionate, which can damage the adrenal glands, cause high blood pressure and diabetes, and severely damage the skin.

Still other products contain another potentially harmful steroid called fluocinonide. All of these steroids can cause acnelike eruptions, stretch marks, skin irritation, loss of skin color, dryness, itching, and hair growth if they are applied over large areas of the body over a prolonged period of time.

Products to Avoid

The U.S. Food and Drug Administration lists unapproved and unauthorized cosmetics and drugs on its website. Government websites are often difficult to navigate. Here's an easy way to find out if a product is on the list: Use the search engine www.google.com. Type in Import Alert IA6641. Click on it and scroll down; you'll find a list of products that probably have familiar names.

Law Enforcement

You may ask the logical question, if these products are illegal, why are they so easy to buy?

The answer appears to be that law enforcement officials in the United States can't keep up with the flood of products that are either smuggled in or simply ordered over the telephone and via the Internet from international sources.

The World Health Organization and African health advocates are pushing countries to ban the manufacture of the mercury-based products. But that hasn't stopped companies from continuing to manufacture and sell the dangerous products. As long as there is a market and people are willing to buy them, the products will be available.

The Bottom Line

It is up to you to be careful about what you buy to use on your skin. Read the labels. Evaluate what the products contain. If they list the ingredients that we mention in this chapter, please don't use them without a doctor's prescription.

Serious health risks are associated with these products. The more you know about them, the safer you will be.

Talk to your friends; let them know what you've discovered. In this way, we hope that you can kill the poison in the grapevine.

Dark Circles

CHAPTER 11

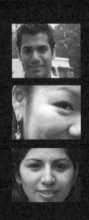

DARK EYES ARE BEAUTIFUL. BUT DARK CIRCLES BELOW THE EYES CAN make you *look* tired and depressed. When your reflection in the mirror is displeasing, you may *feel* depressed.

Margie says she's been avoiding the mirror: "The circles under my eyes are so dark, it looks as if I have taken black paint and painted a mask on. I'm ashamed of how I look and it's causing me to become a recluse. Can you advise me how to remove them?"

We wish we had a magic wand to wave the dark circles away. Unfortunately the answer is a bit more complicated than that.

Why It Happens

There are several causes of dark circles. The simplest reason is rubbing, which can be done unconsciously with your hands or a pair of glasses that rub continuously against the under-eye skin.

But it may also be another one of those family traits embedded in DNA in our cells, passed on through our genes. People from Asia, the Mediterranean, the Middle East, and the Indian subcontinent frequently hand this characteristic down through the generations. And it often shows up in childhood.

Allergies are also an inherited problem that can lead to dark circles. Allergies create inflammation, and the inflammation enlarges the tiny blood vessels beneath your eyes. The swollen blood vessels press against your thin under-eye skin, and the dark color of the blood vessels shows through. As if that weren't bad enough, allergies make your eyes itch. You scratch and rub. That causes trauma and stimulates the cells called melanocytes, which give your skin color. The melanocytes react to the rubbing and scratching by producing darker pigment in that already sensitive area.

Many women get dark circles when they get their periods, are pregnant, or go through menopause, because the hormonal gyrations cause the blood vessels to swell. In addition, lack of sleep, lack of water, too much salt, caffeine, smoking, and using illegal drugs can make the blood vessels swell. Some prescription medications such as diuretics may reduce the fluid in the fat pads of the under-eye area and contribute to dark circles.

The sun is another negative factor. It also stimulates the melanocytes and produces more color. The more the under-eye area is exposed to the sun, the more likely it is that you'll have dark circles.

And then, of course, there is age. As we get older, the thin skin gets even thinner and the blood vessels become more obvious. The under-eye skin also has few oil glands, which makes it more sensitive and less protected.

Remedies
What You Can Do on Your Own
Preventing irritation is the most important thing. Treat your under-eye area like a beautiful piece of silk. Stop rubbing, scratching, or pulling at the skin under the eyes. And begin a management routine that focuses on *gentle* care of the under-eye area. Be careful when you remove your makeup. Use a gentle, unscented makeup remover like Albolene or Pond's cold cream.

Start wearing sun protection immediately. Daily use of sun protection is essential, and is particularly important when treating dark circles. Please think of sunblock as a must-wear every day, all year long, whether or not the sun is out, when you are outside or driving in your car. The sun's rays penetrate your car's windshield. Sun exposure darkens your skin and makes dark circles darker.

We recommend, again, an oil-free sunblock-sunscreen with Parsol 1789, UVA, UVB, and a sun protection factor of 20 to 30, with zinc oxide or titanium dioxide. Make sure that you apply it lightly over the entire eye area. But be careful not to get it in your eyes. Sunblock does sting.

If you have allergies, follow your physician's instructions to treat them; we also recommend gently placing a cool compress over your eyes every day for five to ten minutes. This will help the blood vessels constrict. If they aren't as obvious, the under-eye area won't look as dark.

Regardless of the cause of dark circles, moisturizing is very important. Fifty to 80 percent of our body weight is made up of water. We lose water all of the time as we burn calories and sweat, but water helps plump up our skin, particularly in the under-eye area. You may have noticed that some marathon runners have dark circles under their eyes after a race. They've expended a lot of energy and lost a lot of water. Although there are no concrete studies defining how much water we should drink, the National Research Council suggests that the average man burning 2,900 calories a day needs twelve cups of water, and the average woman needs nine cups of water. Milk, juice, and soup contribute to hydration, but drinking eight to ten glasses of water a day will provide additional moisture for your face and the skin all over your body.

Dr. Downie drinks fifteen glasses of water a day because her skin is very dry. She suggests this example: "If you are one hundred and fifty pounds, you should be drinking eleven glasses of water a day."

Similarly, hydrating eye creams that contain vitamins C and E are good. These vitamins are antioxidants that fight the free-radical oxygen compounds that form naturally in our bodies over the years and cause aging. Vitamin K creams may help to constrict the blood vessels. Because the skin is so thin under the eye, the blood vessels absorb the creams quickly. Even working from the outside, the moisturizers help to plump up the skin by adding moisture and sealing in water. Products with vitamin A may also be helpful because vitamin A helps build the collagen, which naturally gives our skin its nice supple texture.

We have to warn you. You won't be able to cure the problem by taking loads of vitamin A, C, E, or K. You can overdose on vitamins and create other health problems. In addition, topical vitamin A products and retinoids, which are a form of vitamin A, can be very irritating if they are not used sparingly.

Neutrogena Healthy Skin Eye Cream, Avon Lighten Up Undereye Treatment, and Bobbi Brown Hydrating Eye Cream are among the products available for under-eye treatment. Clinique has developed a product especially for men. For Men Eye Treatment Formula is an oil-free moisturizing cream that the company designed to lighten dark circles.

Creams are usually better for normal to dry skin and are easier to use under makeup. Remember, more cream is not necessarily better. Follow the instructions and apply just a small amount so that you don't irritate that sensitive skin. Heavy fragrance can also irritate the skin and make the dark circles worse.

Natural Remedies

Tea bags are a simple way to begin to calm down the tiny blood vessels underneath the eyes. Caffeine in the tea can help constrict the swollen vessels. Apply two cool, moistened bags underneath each eye for a few minutes every night for a week. Depending on the severity of your problem, there may be some improvement.

Taryn sent us an e-mail, saying, "The skin underneath my eyes is not only dark, it is frequently hot. I apply cool cucumber slices to help reduce the heat." Taryn's right. The cucumber slices also moisturize the area, constrict the blood vessels, and calm down the swelling. Like everything else, these natural remedies are beneficial only if you apply them *gently* and consistently.

Over-the-Counter Remedies

Kinerase is a good antiaging and moisturizing product but it is not cheap. You can buy it over the counter, via the Internet, and sometimes in a dermatologist's office. We like it because it is a moisturizing cream with something called N-6 furfuryladenine. Studies have found that this agent helps to slow down aging in the skin cells. It is gentler than many of the acid-based products and is particularly good for the under-eye skin.

A Doctor's Guidance

A dermatologist's guidance may be needed to help manage dark circles. A knowledgeable doctor is likely to recommend a number of things to help.

Chemical Peels

A doctor might suggest a series of chemical peels, using acids that mimic those found in plants, fruits, or milk. We described chemical peels in depth in chapter 7. Asian, olive, and dark skin is particularly sensitive, and although chemical peels can be effective, they must be administered by someone who understands your skin and is experienced at applying chemical peels to people with skin of color.

Prescription Medicines

In addition to the peels, the doctor might prescribe a fading cream. But because this area of your face is so sensitive and your skin is so reactive, it's likely the doctor will ask you to use it less frequently.

EpiQuin Micro is a new product that contains hydroquinone, which helps block an enzyme that makes the skin dark, and a retinol that is released slowly into the skin to prevent irritation.

Glyquin XM and Alustra may also be effective. Both contain hydroquinone, glycolic acid, moisturizing agents, and vitamins C and E. We explain the ingredients in these creams and how they work in chapter 12 on dark blotches and marks. But special care is needed in the under-eye area. It's often a good idea to begin using these creams only once or twice a week and gradually increase to daily use, if your skin isn't irritated.

Makeup

Makeup isn't a remedy. However, while you are treating dark circles, makeup can help you to look and feel better. Dermablend has concealers to match your skin tone. L'Oreal has a cover-up product called HydraFresh Circle Eraser designed for women in their twenties. It contains vitamin C as well as light diffusers that reduce the appearance of circles or lines.

New York makeup artist Alba Luisa Santana recommends Avon Advanced Concealer, which comes in a full range of colors from medium to very dark. She also likes Erno Laszlo stick foundation and pHelitone concealer.

When you choose your foundation or concealer, Alba Luisa suggests mixing it in the palm of your hand with a gentle, hydrating eye cream before you apply it to the under-eye area. For under-eye moisturizing, Alba Luisa likes Clinique's All About Eyes and B-21 from Orlane.

Excellent foundations are also available for skin of color. New York television makeup artist Maryann Muro recommends the I-Iman cosmetic line for skin of color. "I-Iman has sixteen shades of foundation and you can match almost every skin tone. The I Conceal stick concealer is very good for covering up dark circles. This is excellent makeup for dark skin because it never looks ashy or chalky," she says. Maryann recommends experimenting with different colors in the I-Iman line to blend the colors for the under-eye area.

For Asian skin, Maryann suggests foundations from the Shu Uemura cosmetics. "They have a range of colors that blend with Asian skin and really compliment it." In addition she also likes Shiseido foundation, powder, and concealer. In the early twentieth century, Shiseido was the first company to create a powder to match Asian skin tones. Maryann says, "Shiseido products have a great deal of pigment, and they often look flawless on the skin."

In addition to these recommendations, Prescriptives has a color system that includes a range of olive to dark shades. Bobbi Brown makeup also offers darker colors with nice textures.

We do have a warning: it's a good idea to test products on your inner arm before you apply them to the eye area.

The Bottom Line

It isn't always easy or possible to erase dark circles, but it is worth the effort to even out your skin tone. This requires your commitment to carry out a plan devised by either you or your doctor. Getting the best results requires a consistently focused approach.

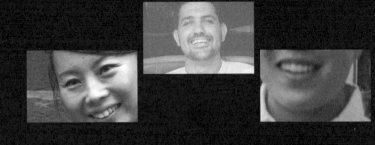

Dark Marks

CHAPTER 12

CERTAIN STRUGGLES SEEM ENDLESS AND UNWINNABLE. ATTEMPTING to fade dark marks is one of them. As you try to even out your skin tone, you may feel as if you're stuck in one of those frustrating dreams in which you're trying to run but your feet won't move. It's a nightmare you share with millions. Many people tell us the dark marks torment them as though they were scars permanently marring their appearance. Although in medical terms dark marks are not scars, they may create emotional scars because they can be so troubling.

The marks appear on people with the darkest skin. Chris e-mailed: "I am an African-American who suffers from complexion-killing dark spots and a feeling of hopelessness about ever having clear skin."

It is also a problem for Asian men and women like Akeiko, who worries: "So many little dark spots have popped on my face in the last few years. Nothing I use does any good."

Dark marks also distress Paula, who, at first glance, appears to have light skin: "I have very bad dark marks and blotches on my skin. On one side of my family, my grandmother was a Native American and my grandfather was African-American. On the other side, my Jewish grandfather was from Russia and my grandmother was from Latin America. I look white and doctors don't seem to know how to treat me. Every time I try something, the dark marks turn into blotches. Is there something I can do?"

With a good skin management plan, and an investment of time and effort, you can even out your skin and fade the dark marks significantly.

Why It Happens

From the time you were young, you've probably noticed that the slightest bruise, scrape, pimple, or wound to your skin leaves a dark mark. Acne usually creates many dark marks. Skin of color is prone to dark marks because of its cellular makeup. The melanocytes, the pigment cells that give your skin color, are very active in dark skin. And whenever the skin is irritated or traumatized in even the smallest way, the melanocytes in the area get revved up. The tyrosinase enzymes in the cells react and create more melanin, or color. You see the results: the dark mark, blotch, or spot. Doctors call this *hyperpigmentation.* Although the marks can drive you crazy, they are generally harmless.

The sun also stimulates the enzymes in the melanocytes. Any mark that you already have on your skin is likely to get darker if exposed to the sun. You don't have to bake in the sun for this to happen. Simply walking down the street, working, or playing outside where sun is reflected from pavement, snow, or water makes you a candidate for a dark mark.

Pregnant women sometimes get dark marks because they are producing more estrogen and progresterone, which stimulate the melanocytes. Similarly, if you are taking birth control pills or using hormone replacement therapy, it is possible you'll develop a dark mark or two. Studies of women using hormone replacement indicate that estrogen is likely to cause the dark marks. Progesterone, however, doesn't.

Remedies

What You Can Do on Your Own

We know that many people feel that they can't afford a visit to a dermatologist or don't have the time for an appointment. But it's a good idea to get the guidance of a board-certified dermatologist or other knowledgeable doctor to help you tackle the problem of dark marks. It's easy to make these dark marks worse.

If you are cruising the stores looking for products, we hope that you'll read chapter 10, "Dangerous Products."

Sun Protection

You have heard this warning before, but it is impossible to say it too often: sun brings out dark marks, and the first line of defense is a sunblock with a sun protection factor of between 20 and 30. We like oil-free sunblock that contains zinc oxide or titanium dioxide and Parsol 1789. These are the ingredients that will provide the strongest protection for your skin. Many companies make sunblocks with these ingredients, and they are available in any drug or beauty supply store. If you are outside, applying sun protection once a day isn't enough. Reapply it every two hours.

Hydroquinone

We are not fans of skin lightening, and we'll urge you to stay away from products that promise to change the color of your skin. But we think that fading a dark mark can improve your appearance without changing the very nature of who you are.

In chapter 10, we discuss dangerous products. Some unscrupulous people often try to take advantage of your desire to fade a dark mark by offering an array of products that may, in the long run, be harmful.

There are, however, products that *do* work. The good products and the dangerous products often contain similar ingredients. Most contain some form of hydroquinone, an agent that blocks tyrosinase, the enzyme that triggers the production of color in the melanoycte cells. Color production slows when the enzyme is blocked. The cells with the dark spots also absorb the hydroquinone and fade. In the United States, you can buy products containing 2 percent hydroquinone over the counter. The problem is that many stores in ethnic neighborhoods carry illegally imported brands with mystery ingredients. These products may claim to contain 2 percent hydroquinone. But the FDA and others aren't sure the labeling is correct.

If you are using a stronger hydroquinone without a doctor's supervision, you run the risk of creating dark and light blotches. Hydroquinone products are regulated tightly or banned in parts of Europe and throughout Asia because studies have shown that high concentrations, and prolonged use, may cause cancer and other health problems.

When you use the correct strength of hydroquinone—again, it is 2 percent if it is sold over the counter—it's important to apply it no more than twice a day in a pea-sized amount over the dark mark. It is also a good idea to test the cream on your skin first. "Some people are allergic to hydroquinone," Dr. Cook-Bolden warns. "When you use a hydroquinone product for the first time, place a small bit in the fold of your arm two or three times a day to test for a reaction. If your skin remains clear after doing this for five days, you probably can use it safely."

OVER-THE-COUNTER PRODUCTS

Ambi Discoloration Fade Cream, Palmer's Skin Success, Esoterica, Porcelana, and Skin Salon Gold are hydroquinone products that appear to be safe.

ALPHA AND BETA HYDROXY PRODUCTS

We described alpha and beta hydroxy acids in chapter 2, "Acne," and chapter 7, "Chemical Peels." We mentioned a number of over-the-counter products that can help to speed up the process of shedding tired skin cells. We like Alpha Hydrox, which is available in most drugstores or beauty supply shops, and Avon Anew, which is easily ordered via the Internet or through an Avon representative. Skin Salon Gold also contains alpha hydroxy acid and can be purchased via the Internet.

But we think that persistent dark marks may need the helping hand of a professional board-certified dermatologist who can administer a series of chemical peels in a strength that works best for you. Please read the chapter on chemical peels where we explain how they work, and the range of options a doctor might choose.

A Doctor's Guidance

Here's where skin care management comes into play. A board-certified dermatologist who is knowledgeable about dark skin will help you establish a program to erase the dark marks and prevent new ones.

Prescription Medicines

After recommending a sunblock, a dermatologist is likely to prescribe a cream containing 4 percent hydroquinone. This is a strength that is usually safe for dark skin, and it is more effective than what's available over the counter. There are several popular products.

Dr. Cook-Bolden recommends Glyquin XM. It contains 4 percent hydroquinone, glycolic acid, one of the alpha hydroxy acids, moisturizing agents, and antioxidant vitamins C and E to help fight the oxygen compounds that form in your body and cause aging.

Dr. Downie likes to prescribe Lustra-AF, which contains 4 percent hydroquinone, vitamins C and E, glycolic acid, and moisturizing agents, as well as Parsol 1789, which helps screen the sun's rays. "This gives you an additional benefit. You can apply the cream in the morning and start out with sun protection. That's one of the reasons I like to prescribe it," she says.

If the dark marks are persistent, the dermatologist might prescribe Alustra, which is a favorite of both Dr. Downie and Dr. Cook-Bolden. Alustra contains 4 percent hydroquinone as well as retinol, which is a vitamin A derivative that helps to boost the collagen in the skin, dry clogged pores, and speed the natural peeling process of dead skin cells. It also contains vitamins C and E and glycerin, which attracts moisture to the skin.

Similarly, Tri-Luma Cream is a prescription medicine combining several therapies. Dr. Downie says, "I like this very much because it includes four percent hydroquinone, a topical steroid, and tretinoin—a vitamin A derivative. The combination makes it extremely potent, and it can be helpful if your dark marks are resistant to everything else."

But because it contains a steroid that can thin the skin too much, or potentially cause acne, Tri-Luma should be used for a limited time. Depending on how your skin responds, your doctor may suggest that you use it every day for three to six months and then cut back to once a week for another three to six months.

A relatively new product called EpiQuin Micro has delivered promising results. It contains 4 percent hydroquinone and retinol. A special formulation allows the ingredients to seep slowly into the skin to prevent irritation.

The doctor may prescribe Retin-A Micro or Tazorac, full-strength retinoids that speed the exfoliation of dead skin cells and consequently help to even out skin color. Research has shown that both Retin-A Micro and Tazorac may also lighten the skin.

A series of chemical peels, which remove layers of dead skin cells, can also be a central part of the treatment plan. We explain chemical peels in chapter 7. They are extremely effective for evening out skin tone and creating a clear complexion because they help the hyroquinone seep into the deep skin cells. Chemical peels and retinoids work very well together to help reduce dark marks. One chemical peel is usually not enough. We like to apply a chemical peel every two to four weeks over a period of several months to a year. And it may take that long before you see a real difference.

Microdermabrasion is also helpful. A series of microdermabrasion sessions can remove layers of dead skin and increase the penetration of hydroquinone. It's a good idea to alternate microdermabrasion therapy with chemical peels every two to four weeks.

Makeup

Because getting results takes time, you may want to use makeup to camouflage the dark marks while treating them. Dermablend provides excellent coverage and comes in a range of darker colors. The I-Iman makeup line is designed for skin of color. There are sixteen shades suited to skin of color from the lightest skin to the darkest. And the I Conceal coverage stick may be able to cover the dark marks. This line is a favorite of television makeup artist Maryann Muro who says, "The I-Iman line has tones of orange in the products. The foundations and concealers don't make dark skin look chalky or ashy. It gives you a smooth look without that masklike effect."

For Asian skin, Maryann prefers the Shiseido and Shu Uemura lines. Both make foundations, powder, and concealers that match a range of Asian skin tones. "Shu Uemura makes an excellent foundation," she says. "And Shiseido has a variety of formulations so you can experiment and see which feels most comfortable on your skin."

MAC, Avon, Bobbi Brown, and Prescriptives also have foundations in darker shades.

The Bottom Line

Dark marks may appear overnight, but unfortunately you can't eliminate them that quickly. You need to commit to a program of skin care and stick with it. It is possible to have an even skin tone and defeat dark marks, but only if you protect yourself from the sun and treat blemishes and injuries to the skin quickly and correctly. Please be patient with your skin. Treat it with respect. And give it the time it needs to renew itself. Remember, go *gently*.

Dry Skin
CHAPTER 13

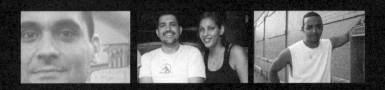

BEFORE YOU TURN THE PAGE, THINK ABOUT THIS: BEAUTIFUL SKIN OF any color is supple, soft, and feels good to the touch. Experts talk about hydration and lubrication. What they mean is that we need water to keep our skin moist. It is the water in our bodies that helps skin to look healthy.

If your skin itches and looks patchy, if you can see the outlines of skin cells, if you are peeling and you're not trying to exfoliate, these are signs that your skin is crying out for attention. Your skin is letting you know that it's too dry.

Dry skin can be dramatically improved. The more water you drink and the more moisture you apply to your skin, the healthier your skin will look and feel. If you are prone to dry skin, this can be a lifelong management issue. Moisturizers must be applied daily. Sometimes, you'll have to apply moisturizers more frequently, especially when it's cold or dry outside.

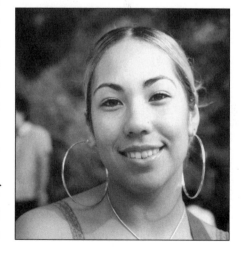

Dr. Cook-Bolden says, "Moisturizing three times a day can really help. It may sound like a tough job, but if you apply moisturizer in the morning before you dress, when you return home from work or school, and before you go to bed at night, you can counteract the dryness."

Most moisturizers protect your skin by sealing in the moisture that's already there. When you apply a moisturizer, your skin feels smooth. As the body absorbs this moisturizer, a slight, temporary swelling occurs that makes the surface skin cells look better.

There are also moisturizers that contain humectants. Humectants attract water when you put them on your skin. Dr. Cook-Bolden says, "For very dry skin, moisturizers with humectants are the best. They really add water to your skin."

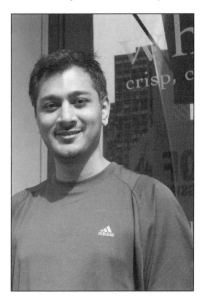

This means that it's a good idea to read the labels of the moisturizers. Ideally, you should look for a humectant moisturizer that contains one or more humectants including: glycerin, sorbitol, urea, alpha hydroxy acids. Lactic acid is especially effective. LAC-HYDRIN and AmLactin are two good over-the-counter moisturizers containing lactic acid.

There are other effective moisturizers, and we offer a full review of these products in chapter 3 on ashy skin.

We also find that adding moisture to the air helps to relieve dry skin. It may be a good idea to place a shallow pan of water near a radiator in the winter months. Humidifiers are also effective. Dr. Downie has suffered with dry skin since she was child. "I find that using a humidifier in my bedroom helps tremendously. It keeps the air moist and it adds moisture to my skin," she says.

Wind, cold, and the sun also contribute to dry skin. Using extra moisturizer during cold and windy months will help, and wearing sun protection can make a huge difference. As we've said before, we recommend a sunblock with Parsol 1789, UVA and UVB protection, zinc oxide or titanium oxide, and a sun protection factor of 20 to 30. See also chapter 3, "Ashy Skin."

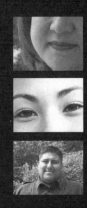

Eczema

CHAPTER 14

ANYONE WHO SUFFERS FROM ECZEMA KNOWS HOW UNCOMFORTABLE
and distressing it can be. Dr. Downie has struggled with eczema since
she was a toddler. "My mother is a pediatrician, and she first noticed it
on my legs and arms when I was about a year old," she says.

Eczema is one of the most common skin diseases. Doctors use the
term *eczema* to describe a number of skin irritations that look alike
and are usually very itchy. Many of these conditions begin in infancy.
A doctor may tell you that it is also known as *atopic dermatitis.*

Like Dr. Downie's mom, parents are in a frustrating search for
remedies. Victoria wrote to us asking for help for her daughter: "Ever
since she was born, my daughter has had a problem with her skin. At
the age of two, she was diagnosed with eczema. I've tried everything.
Nothing seems to work."

There's no cure for eczema, but it can be managed.

Why It Happens

Most eczema is thought to be hereditary. If you or your child suffer
from eczema, it's likely that it's preprogrammed in your DNA.
Eczema is also thought to be linked to allergies, including hay fever.
People who have asthma are also eczema-prone. Eczema sufferers
have extremely sensitive skin. They are likely to be far more susceptible to mild skin irritations and stress-related skin disorders than oth-

ers. Some researchers think stress may trigger eczema, but they haven't yet been able to make the scientific link.

Hypersensitivity to chemicals, detergents, food, and nickel can cause eczema. Research suggests that babies may develop eczema in reaction to infant formula. Ingredients in some baby wipes may also aggravate eczema. To be on the safe side, you may want to use a very mild cleanser such as Cetaphil on a damp paper towel instead of a packaged wipe.

One type of eczema appears in babies between the ages six months and two years. Dr. Cook-Bolden says, "It is particularly upsetting for parents because the eczema can look so bad and we know that you really want to help your baby."

The eczema can develop anywhere on the body but usually forms on a baby's forehead, cheeks or scalp, elbows, or knees, and then moves to the folds of the arms and legs.

Often, there's an itchy, oozing rash that may get crusty. Eczema is unlikely to hurt, but it does itch. "Infants don't have the reflex to scratch. So you've got to keep it clean and soothe it for them," Dr. Cook-Bolden says.

If the eczema is rubbed or scratched, particularly as children get older, it often becomes so raw that it is easily infected, and that may lead to scarring.

Over time, eczema changes slightly. The oozing may stop, and the patch of eczema may disappear from the cheeks and elbows and move to the folds of the legs and arms. There are likely to be dry, itchy, red or brown patches.

The news here is moderately hopeful. Research indicates that 60 to 70 percent of children who have eczema seem to outgrow it by the time they reach their teens.

Dr. Downie, however, says, "I certainly didn't outgrow my eczema. It's gotten a lot better. But I still have patches of it on the back of my neck."

In adults, eczema is often dry and itchy. The skin frequently breaks out into raw, bleeding patches. Older people who develop eczema on their legs may have a circulatory problem that requires medical attention.

This may all sound familiar and grim to you, but there really is a way to stay on top of it and soothe your skin.

Remedies

What You Can Do on Your Own

You can control the eczema by the way you treat the skin every minute of every day.

Try not to scratch, and try to keep your child from scratching. It may sound like obvious advice, but scratching makes things so much worse. Maintaining short nails is a good way to prevent a child, or yourself, from doing real damage.

When the itching is very bad, an oral antihistamine like Benadryl might help. You want to make sure that you are using the right dose.

Cool baths or showers help. Use a gentle soap such as Dove, Neutrogena, or Aveeno Body Wash, Skin Relief, Fragrance Free. Or try a bath with Aveeno Dry Skin (Oilated) Formula Bath Treatment. The mineral oil in the product can be very soothing. Apply moisturizers after bathing or washing while the skin is still damp. This helps to seal in the moisture. You may have to apply moisturizer many times throughout the day, so try carrying a small tube of moisturizer with you.

The moisturizers we like best include Cetaphil, Curel, Eucerin, Lubriderm, SBR Lipocream, Aquaphor Healing Ointment, Vanicream, and Jergens Ash Relief. These are thick, soothing lotions and creams that can make you feel better and improve the appearance of your skin.

Another way to calm the itching is to gently place a damp washcloth or piece of gauze over the eczema. Dr. Downie gets relief for her eczema by applying an ice cube directly on the spot and then applying a moisturizer immediately after removing the ice cube.

Fabrics that surround you are also a big factor. What you wear and what you sit on and sleep under have an effect on sensitive skin. Make sure that anything that touches your skin or your child's skin isn't too tight, doesn't rub, and feels soft. Cotton, for example, is much gentler than wool, which can make the skin itch.

Nickel can also be an irritant. Clothing manufacturers frequently use nickel for fasteners, snaps, and zippers. Dr. Downie had a patch of eczema near her belly button when she was a teenager. The snaps and zippers on her jeans always made the eczema worse. "I realized that I had to cover the zippers and snaps on my jeans if I wanted to wear them. I coated them with two coats of clear nail polish, and it worked. The nickel wasn't directly on my skin, and it wasn't irritated," she says. Often, it is necessary to avoid metal snaps, zippers, and fasteners and switch to buttons and elastic.

Anyone with eczema is environmentally sensitive. Very hot and very cold temperatures aggravate the eczema. Try to control your climate at home and avoid placing yourself or child in sweaty clothes or situations. Sweat may make the eczema worse.

Because chemicals are thought to trigger eczema, be careful about what gets on the skin. Don't stop living, but make sure you wash harsh things off your skin as soon as possible. This includes household cleaners and chlorine from swimming pools.

We don't want to discourage you from exercising. Stress, we think, is a factor in eczema flare-ups, and regular exercise can help you to manage stress. Just remember that you need to shower carefully after exercising to wash off any perspiration.

Prescription Medicines

Doctors want to treat the eczema, but we don't want to overprescribe potentially dangerous medication. In some cases, we will prescribe a topical steroid for a limited period. We've described the possibly harmful effects they can have with prolonged use. Sometimes a doctor will prescribe a steroid to be applied to the skin for two to four weeks; only with a doctor's advice should the steroid cream be used for longer periods.

There are two new, nonsteroid prescription medications called *immune modulators* that work on the immune system and are showing positive results in the treatment of eczema. One is called Protopic and the other is Elidel.

Antihistamines like Atarax or the generic hydroxyzine, Benadryl, Clarinex, Claritin, Zyrtec, and Doxepin in low doses can also be a valuable part of the treatment for eczema. They help decrease the itching.

The Bottom Line

Finding small ways to manage your skin or your child's skin may require a little creativity. Some things may work better than others on your skin. Experiment with one thing at a time. Keep a list of things that make the eczema flare up and try to avoid them. In addition, keep a supply of soothing lotions and creams in your home, in your hand-bag, or on your desk at work. Put a tube of moisturizer in your child's backpack as he or she goes to school. You can make your life, and your child's life, more comfortable until scientists discover something that really works to cure eczema.

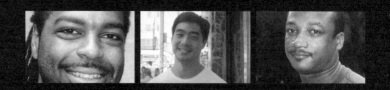

Facial Hair—Men

CHAPTER 15

MOST MEN TAKE FACIAL HAIR FOR GRANTED. IT'S A SYMBOL OF masculinity. You mature, and your hair grows. You begin to shave and the hair is gone until the stubble signals that the hair is on its way back. But for many men, especially African-Americans, Caribbean-Americans, and men of Middle Eastern and Latin American descent, it is not as simple as that. You may be prone to developing razor bumps, or ingrown hairs, or, in medical terms, *pseudofolliculitis barbae*.

This is a medical condition that afflicts people with curly hair. Like other medical problems involving dark skin, there hasn't been a great deal of research on ingrown hairs. But it's estimated that at least 80 percent of all African-American men suffer from razor bumps.

Razor bumps develop anywhere hair is shaved, tweezed, or waxed. The problem occurs most frequently on the face. Men young and old tell us about painful attempts to pick or shave away the ingrown hairs, which develop into painful, inflamed bumps that resemble acne. And to compound the problem, when the bumps go away they leave a great deal of discoloration.

> **FACT:** *It's estimated that at least 80 percent of all African-American men suffer from razor bumps.*

Paul's e-mail tells a familiar story: "I have a terrible time shaving. First, I have ingrown hairs. My number two concern is the dark spots.

My skin looks awful and it's embarrassing. People at work keep asking, 'What's wrong with your skin?'"

Even if you manage to live with the discomfort, the terrible discoloration draws unwanted attention. Dr. Downie says, "The skin where you shave can become two to three shades darker than the rest of the skin. The darkness on the neck really stands out. Shaving is so painful that many of my patients ask for excuse notes. They want me to tell their supervisors that they can only shave two or three times a week. And these are grown men!"

We understand how difficult this problem can be. If you have a corporate or government job, you are generally expected to be clean-shaven. Historically, it has been a problem in the military; men were discharged from the service when they refused to shave.

Razor bumps can be eased in a variety of ways, and Dr. Cook-Bolden is particularly enthusiastic about laser treatments. "Fortunately we are revolutionizing the treatment of razor bumps," Dr. Cook-Bolden says. "The development of laser technology has allowed us to tackle the problem of pseudofolliculitis barbae by almost painlessly removing hair and improving the condition of the skin."

Why It Happens

It may help to understand why you get razor bumps. Very curly, coiled hair curves as it comes out of the scalp, face, or neck. When curly hair is cut, there's a knifelike point at the end. That point can easily bend back and dig into the skin. Once the hair penetrates the skin, the body reacts to what it now considers a "foreign body." The reaction causes inflammation, making a razor bump. A bump is often painful and itchy and when you pick at it, it gets worse.

We know that you may want to take a needle to try to dig out the hair. Darren wrote to us saying, "I sterilize a needle by putting it to the flame of a lighter and dipping it in alcohol, but I still get infected."

Trying to pick out the hair can create infections and scars.

Remedies
What You Can Do on Your Own

Changing the way you shave is the first step. Shaving immediately after you take a shower or bath makes a differ- ence. Having soft, moist skin will make it easier to shave. Be gentle. Don't pull or stretch the skin.

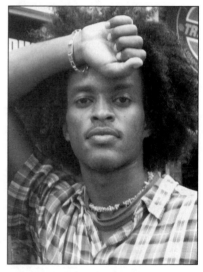

The shaving cream you use is impor- tant. Creams with scents can easily irritate the skin. We like Aveeno Shave Gel. It is a rich, smooth gel that contains oatmeal and allantoin, an agent that moisturizes and soothes damaged skin and is fragrance-free. Neutrogena Razor Defense is also a rich, thick gel that softens the skin and hair with- out being greasy or irritating. Glytone Seri- ous Shave Cream is another good product. It contains glycolic acid, which helps to speed the shedding of dead skin cells and smooth the skin.

The type of razor that you use can also reduce the possibility of ingrown hairs. Doctors have a difference of opinion here.

Dr. Downie recommends a triple-edged razor. "You get a closer shave. And the hairs in the beard area don't form stubble. They don't get a chance to turn back into the skin." She particularly likes the Mach3Turbo from Gillette.

But Dr. Cook-Bolden thinks the triple-edged razor may be too much of a good thing. She says, "When the first blade cuts the hair, it makes a sharp point. The action of the second and third blades may put too much pressure on the hair and cause it to snap back and curl under the skin to form razor bumps." She points out, "Not all men will react the same way. It's important to find the razor that gives you the best result and does the least harm."

Many men like to use an electric razor because they think it decreases the razor bumps. If you have very sensitive skin, this may help you get a smooth shave. But using an electric razor doesn't necessarily guarantee that you will be razor bump–free.

Shaving is so personal. And the tools you use really depend on your individual needs. But the object should always be to get a close shave without allowing the hairs to curl back into the skin.

If one type of razor doesn't work for you, experiment with another. You may be surprised by something that you haven't tried before.

TIP: *It's really a bad idea to use fragrant aftershave lotions. Scent irritates the skin. Instead, try an oil-free moisturizer that won't clog your pores.*

If you are using a nonelectric razor, the blade or blades must be sharp and fresh. Discard the cartridge or disposable razor after you've used it a few times, and change to a new one. Dull blades drag against the skin. They increase the possibility that the hair will curl back into the skin.

Make sure that you shave in the direction in which your hair grows, and that you only shave an area once. Repeatedly shaving a section increases the possibility that you'll create a razor bump.

It's really a bad idea to use fragrant aftershave lotions. Scent irritates the skin. Instead, try an oil-free moisturizer that won't clog your pores. We like Neutrogena Moisture and Bobbi Brown Soothing Face Tonic containing green tea and glycerine to attract moisture and soothe the skin. Eucerin Renewal Alpha Hydroxy Lotion-For Face may be a good moisturizer to use after shaving when your face is completely dry; applying the alpha hydroxy product to your wet skin directly after shaving may irritate it.

Calming the Irritation

Your total skin care program is important. For someone who is prone to razor bumps, it is more than a matter of shaving or washing your face. A management plan is required to keep the razor bumps and the problems that come with them under control.

Sun protection is critical in the campaign to conquer the discoloration caused by razor bumps. Sunlight will make the dark marks even darker. We continue to recommend an oil-free sunblock with Parsol 1789, UVA and UVB protection, and a sun protection factor of 20 to 30, preferably with zinc oxide or titanium dioxide.

You may have heard women talk about alpha and beta hydroxy acids. In earlier chapters, we explain that these acids, which are contained in a variety of washes, creams, and chemical peels, help slough off dead skin, calm inflamed acne bumps, and improve overall skin texture. They also will decrease the inflammation from razor bumps, improve the texture of your skin, and decrease discoloration.

You can buy products such as Aqua Glycolic or Alpha Hydrox in a drugstore, or Avon Anew via the Internet or through an Avon representative. Neutrogena's Razor Defense Lotion is also effective. Tend

Skin is a popular product that is effective for many men. It contains beta hydroxy or salicylic acid. Before applying any of these products to your face, test a small amount in the fold of your arm to see how your skin reacts. When you use one of these products, please don't rub or scrub your skin. Grainy scrubs are likely to be irritating. No amount of scrubbing will make the razor bumps go away.

If proper shaving and glycolic washes don't help, it may be necessary to see a dermatologist who can design a good skin management program especially for you.

A Doctor's Guidance

In addition to reviewing the way you shave and how you care for your skin at home, the doctor may recommend a series of chemical peels, a process we describe in chapter 7.

Chemical peels remove the top layers of your dead skin cells and eliminate the roughness that the razor bumps have created on the surface. The peels also help to even out your skin tone if the skin is badly discolored by the bumps. They also soothe the razor bumps by reducing the inflammation and boosting the skin's natural collagen, which improves the overall texture of your skin.

Prescription Medicines

As part of your plan, consider a morning and evening routine. Dr. Downie asks her patients to use a topical antibiotic gel as well as the glycolic washes in the morning. She also prescribes a 4 percent hydroquinone to lighten the dark spots. "Sometimes I prescribe a higher strength, and I like men to use it in the morning and in the evening," she says.

If your skin can tolerate it, your doctor might recommend benzoyl peroxide for evening use to reduce bacteria. We would alternate use of the benzoyl peroxide with a retinoid to heal the razor bumps and speed the shedding of the dark and damaged skin. The retinoids also stimulate your skin's natural collagen.

Dr. Cook-Bolden uses a slightly different combination therapy to treat razor bumps. "I like the topical antibiotic benzoyl peroxide gels such as Benzamycin and Benzaclin. I recommend that you use one of these antibiotic gels in the morning. You have the benefit of two remedies in one product. Benzamycin also comes as individually packaged wipes, which are easy and convenient to use. I prescribe the antibiotic gel along with a retinoid like Retin-A Micro, Differin, or Tazorac and a topical hydroquinoine cream to even the skin color. Both the retinoid and the hydroquinone cream are applied in a pea-size amount every night and together they really make a difference."

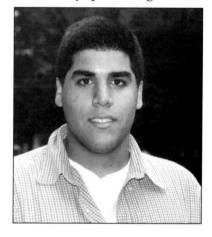

For moderate or severe bumps, the doctor might prescribe an oral antibiotic like doxycycline-Doryx or minocycline-Dynacin. We describe the side effects and contraindications of strong, oral antibiotics in chapter 2 on acne.

When razor bumps are painful, doctors usually inject a small amount of a steroid directly into the worst bumps to ease the inflammation. Or the doctor might prescribe a mild steroid cream to apply to the bumps for no more than two weeks.

Laser Hair Removal

Many people have the same question Charles asked: "Is it safe to have laser hair removal treatments on my face? I'm a dark-skinned man with very bad razor bumps and nothing seems to work. I'm really desperate."

In recent years, new lasers have been designed that are safe for use on skin of color. When a qualified dermatologist or plastic surgeon uses the appropriate laser, the results are usually excellent. Dr. Cook-Bolden has studied the effectiveness of the Lightsheer Diode laser for treatment of pseudofolliculitis barbae and found that when using the appropriate laser, hair was removed, inflammation decreased, and the skin became smoother and softer in most cases.

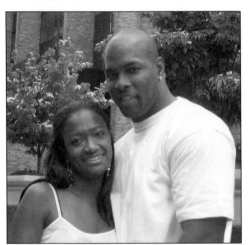

Dr. Cook-Bolden's study involved a laser manufactured by one company. There are also other safe, effective lasers made by a number of manufacturers. In addition, nonlaser light treatment has been effective in treating razor bumps and removing hair. Both laser and light treatments are now standard medical practice for the treatment of pseudofolliculitis barbae. We explain details of laser and light procedures more fully in chapter 19 on hair removal.

COST

The price of laser and light treatments will vary depending on the skill of the doctor and where you live. Many doctors will create a package price for a series of treatments. The cost may range from $400 for a single treatment to $5,000 for a series of treatments that may be administered over the course of a year or more.

The Bottom Line

Although treating the bumps is necessary to ease the inflammation and reduce the pain, sometimes removing the hair that causes the bumps is the best answer. You may not want to remove all your facial hair, but it is possible to remove the hair in the areas that are the most irritated. Chapter 19 provides a full explanation of hair removal.

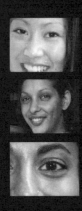

Facial Hair—Women

CHAPTER 16

HATSHEPSUT, THE GREAT FEMALE PHARAOH OF EGYPT IN THE fifteenth century B.C. declared herself both king and queen. To ensure that she was taken seriously, she often wore the ceremonial clothes of a man, including a beard made of gold. As far as we know, underneath the false beard, she had smooth and beautiful skin free of facial hair.

A false beard is one thing. Real facial hair is something else. Facial hair can be a big problem for many women with Asian, olive, and dark skin. Most of us have some hair on our faces, but millions have far more than their fair share. One in six American women is thought to have excess facial hair. Women whose families are from the Mediterranean region and the Indian subcontinent and some African-American, Caribbean-American, and Latina women are the most likely to suffer from the problem.

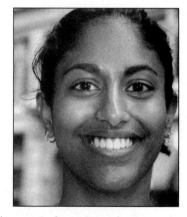

Deandra wrote to us complaining that she has been fighting facial hair for a good part of her thirty-two years. She said: "Unfortunately, I have been cursed with excessive hair growth on my chin and neck. I have tried waxing, shaving, and all types of creams to remove the hair. But it has left bad scarring on my neck."

By the time a woman feels desperate enough to write to us or to see a doctor, she has usually tweezed, waxed, and shaved and, like Deandra, ends up miserable.

Dr. Downie says, "Women come in crying. They say, 'I've tried everything and I still hear people whisper that I look like a man.' It is very frustrating for them."

Darlene's letter to us could have been written by many women we know: "I'm thirty years old and desperate. I want to look like a woman, but I have facial hair on my chin and my cheeks. I've been shaving and tweezing. It seems to have done more harm than good. I have a rough beard and dark marks where I've tweezed. I guess I have more male hormones than I should. I can never go out without tons of makeup."

Jana brought up another problem that women share with men when she wrote, "I have hair on my chin. And I tweeze. Sometimes I get ingrown hairs that hurt and I get dark spots."

Ingrown hairs are very common among women with curly hair. Like razor bumps, ingrown hairs are the medical condition called pseudofolliculitis barbae. Women and men with curly, coiled hair experience the same problem. When you shave, tweeze, or cut your facial hair, you can create a sharp end. Because your hair is curly, it can bend back into the skin and create inflammation, which creates the bump.

The causes of female facial hair are complicated, and those with the condition may require additional medical attention. It helps to have an understanding of what's going on inside of you.

Why It Happens

We need to make an important distinction about women's facial hair. Any facial hair is upsetting and can be a challenge to treat. Many women have light facial hair, which is not unusual. It may appear as a faint shadow on the upper lip, on the jaw line, or as a few hairs on the chin.

This minor to moderate facial hair is hereditary and relatively easy to manage.

Some women, however, develop more than the normal amount. Many women develop a beardlike growth of thick and persistent hairs. The same kind of hair usually appears on the back, on the buttocks, around the nipples, on the lower abdomen, and on the inner thighs. It doesn't look feminine, and it can be hugely embarrassing and upsetting. We know that if you are a woman who suffers from this hair growth, you may be reluctant to talk about it.

Carmen sent us an e-mail about her fear of dating: "Who'd date someone who looks like a woman from the neck down but has a man's face? They might think that I was going through some sort of treatment to become a woman. I'm not. This is me. Please help."

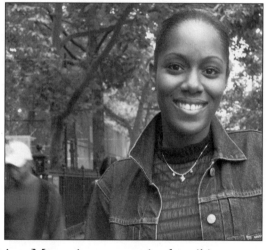

"People can be very insensitive. My patients come in describing how people make fun of them because they have stubble on the cheeks from shaving," Dr. Cook-Bolden says.

Some women can take small comfort in the fact that excess facial hair is a family trait. Male and female relatives are likely to have more hair than the average person. In these families there is usually just a predisposition to excess hair growth, and no serious medical problem.

Hormones

When there is a problem, it may be the result of an hormonal imbalance. You may have first noticed facial hair after you reached puberty. That early hair was probably finely textured and didn't pose much of a problem, at least not at first. But as you got older the hair got coarser, thicker, and more problematic. When this happens, women automatically assume that they're overly endowed with male hormones, which could in fact be the case.

All women naturally produce testosterone, but some women produce higher levels of it and some even produce an excess amount. Testosterone stimulates hair growth. If you have a predisposition to excess hair, the slightest elevation of your testosterone level will make the hair grow. And facial hair is often accompanied by acne, because high levels of testosterone can start the acne cycle. It begins as testosterone stimulates the glands. They produce more oil, which clogs the pores and creates a climate for bacteria to form. The bacteria buildup leads to inflammation and acne eruptions. We provide a full description of the acne cycle in chapter 2.

But why are testosterone levels increased in the first place? That's a good question requiring a little bit of medical sleuthing.

Weight

A healthy, balanced diet helps keep the hormones in check. If excess facial hair appears suddenly, it is possible that it may be connected to what you are eating and to your weight.

Hormones are stored in fat. When you are overweight, you may be storing too many hormones. Excessive hormones, including testosterone, release into your system and stimulate the hair growth.

Your hormones may also be upset if you are on the other end of the scale. If you've had sudden weight loss, or are otherwise underweight, you may have an eating disorder called *anorexia nervosa*, which makes you shun food. Anorexia interrupts and can stop the menstrual cycle. Without

> **FACT:** *A healthy, balanced diet helps keep the hormones in check. If excess facial hair appears suddenly, it is possible that it may be connected to what you are eating and to your weight.*

the production of female hormones, the testosterone can take over and produce more hair. If you are suffering from anorexia nervosa, you may have very fine, thin hair on your cheeks and chest.

Oral Contraceptives

It is possible that the formulation of the oral contraceptive that you're using is upsetting your hormonal balance. Oral contraceptives are also frequently prescribed to control the male hormones and prevent excess hair growth. Your gynecologist or family physician can help you find the right formula for you.

Adrenal and Pituitary Glands

When the answers aren't obvious, as they so often aren't, doctors will conduct blood tests. It is possible that there may be a problem in either your adrenal or pituitary gland. Both glands naturally produce testosterone. When either gland produces too much, it is a signal that something is wrong.

A series of routine blood tests can help pinpoint the problem. If your dermatologist discovers the problem, she or he will recommend that you see your family physician or a specialist to treat the medical condition.

Ovarian Cysts

Excess facial hair is also linked to a hormonal imbalance caused by ovarian cysts. And if the dermatologist has conducted blood tests to rule out other issues, he or she will suggest that you see your gynecologist or family physician for treatment of the underlying problem.

Dr. Cook-Bolden advises, "If there's a medical condition that is causing the facial hair, it's important to treat it while you are working on the remedies to cosmetically eliminate the hair. Solving the basic problem will help make the cosmetic treatments more effective."

Remedies

Excess facial hair is a big enough problem. We don't want to make your life more complicated. If you are shaving, waxing, or tweezing and that works for you—it's fine. Please remember to moisturize after you

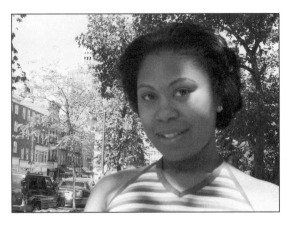

remove the hair. You want to be kind to the skin. If you have razor bumps, calm them down with the treatments we've suggested (see pages 139–143). You may need to see a board-certified dermatologist for help. If the doctor is knowledgeable about skin of color, he or she can set up a program that will control the bumps and possibly remove the hair without causing irritation.

There are a number of effective hair removal methods, including laser hair removal. Because these hair removal techniques can be used by both men and women and on all areas of the body, we'll talk about them in chapter 19 on hair removal.

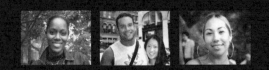

Hair Care and Hair Loss

GREAT HAIR MAKES A BIG DIFFERENCE IN THE WAY YOU LOOK AND IN the way that people look at you. We're among the many people who agonize over our hair, spending hundreds of hours and billions of dollars on hair products each year as we try to make the most of what we have.

This isn't just a women's issue. Increasingly, men are using hairstyling techniques that women have traditionally called their own. The problem is that many of the things that we do to improve the appearance of the hair can damage it, and we don't see the consequences until much later.

We hear from many women who notice sudden hair breakage, bald patches, and thinning hairlines.

Kendra e-mailed us about her problem: "I'm losing my hair around my temples. My hair line practically starts at my ears. I would like to know if there is something that I can do to correct this."

We see the same receding hairline pattern in many women, young and old, whose hair has been mistreated. In a recent study on female hair loss, Dr. Cook-Bolden found that grooming practices are the root cause. And some of these

FACT: *The troubling fact is that African-American, Caribbean-American, and Latina women, and others with tightly coiled curly hair are more likely than people with straight hair to experience hair loss because of their hairstyling methods.*

traditional styling practices cause hair loss in children as young as five years old. The troubling fact is that African-American, Caribbean-American, and Latina women, and others with tightly coiled curly hair are more likely than people with straight hair to experience hair loss because of their hairstyling methods.

"From as far back as I can remember, my mother and my great-aunt braided my hair so tight that I sometimes got headaches," Dr. Downie recalls. "I have almond-shaped eyes. And they would pull my hair back so that the skin stretched and made my eyes turn up at the corners. I'm convinced that's why today I have a thin hair line. And it's why, whenever I see a patient with a child whose hair is too tight, I warn them that it may be next to impossible to get the hair back once the hair loss begins."

FACT: *The quest for perfect hair contributes to breakage and hair loss. If you are otherwise healthy and are torturing your hair, and most of us do, you're likely to have a problem. Coloring, perming, straightening, adding chemicals to your hair, and applying heat via a blow-dryer or curling iron, damages the hair.*

But you don't have to have tightly coiled hair to have a problem. Asian women have thicker, coarser hair than most other women, and thickness doesn't protect the hair from damage. Asian women pull their hair back and use harsh chemicals to color, perm, and straighten their hair, and new chemical procedures including thermal straightening have been developed in Asia.

New York hairstylist Young Choo of the Pierre Michele salon says, "Many Asian women use chemicals to soften their hair as well as to perm or straighten it. Japanese, or thermal, hair straightening has become very popular. Someone looking at Asian hair may think it is straight. But in fact, there are subtle differences. Many people have slightly wavy hair, and some women straighten because they want a smoother, sleeker look. If the straightening is done properly, the hair has more bounce and needs very little other styling help."

The quest for perfect hair contributes to breakage and hair loss.

Lisa e-mailed about hair breakage: "I have dark Asian hair. I've been adding highlights and straightening it for a few years. Now I notice that my ends are breaking. And a lot of hair ends up in the sink when I comb my hair. Can I stop this?"

Regardless of the type of hair you have, you can stop hair breakage and most hair loss if you treat your hair *gently*. Understanding how hair grows and appropriate ways to care for your hair on a regular basis may help to prevent further damage.

Why It Happens
About Your Hair

Each hair begins life as a long narrow cell in the dermis—below the top layers of your skin. The type of hair, the color, and the pattern in which it grows is regulated by your DNA. Like everything else in your body, your genes determine what your hair will look like and whether it will be tightly coiled, curly, or straight.

The color is also determined by your DNA. The melanocyte cells produce pigment and transfer the color to the hair cells. The more pigment cells there are, the darker the hair will be. In addition, if your melanocyte cells produce more eumelanin, you'll have darker hair, and if they produce more phenomelanin, you'll have lighter hair. Many people have a little bit of both types of color pigment.

As cells multiply in the dermis and it gets crowded, older cells are pushed upward. Specialized hair cells fill with the protein keratin and pile up on one another. As they collect, the cells harden and die. Healthy cells continue to push them up out of the scalp. If your hair is very curly, it curves as it comes out of the scalp.

The keratin that hardens the hair follicle also makes it strong. Amino acids in the keratin give the hair the resistance it needs to withstand most of the things you do to it and to protect it from the environment.

In a healthy scalp, new hair follicles are always being pushed out. Hair usually grows at the rate of about one-quarter to half an inch each month. Asians typically have the fewest hairs, with about 90,000 hair follicles on the scalp. People of African descent have about 120,000 hair follicles, and Caucasians have 100,000 to 150,000, depending on the color. Redheads have the fewest hairs, and blondes have the most.

The hairs grow in cycles, and it is natural to shed some. An average healthy adult can lose a hundred to two hundred hairs a day. If you suddenly notice hair falling out, Dr. Downie suggests keeping track of how many hairs you're losing. "If your hair loss jumps from thirty to ninety hairs a day and this continues for six months or more, it is probable that you're experiencing treatable hair loss," she says.

Heredity

Serious hair loss in men and women can be a family trait. Either side of your family could have passed it on to you. Both men and women lose their hair. Male pattern baldness affects more men than women, but women experience it as well, and over half the adult population has some hair loss by the time they reach their fifties. The hair loss may even begin after you hit puberty, although you may not notice the thinning until you're in your twenties.

Hormones

Your hormones contribute to hair growth and hair loss. When androgen and estrogen levels change as you get older, hair follicles shrink and the hair doesn't grow as much as it once did.

Hormone levels also fluctuate during and after pregnancy, and your hair-growth pattern may change. You may have thicker hair when you are pregnant, and then start to lose hair suddenly after giving birth. Karen e-mailed: "After I gave birth and came home from the hospital, I didn't do anything to my hair. I'm embarrassed to admit this, but I didn't even wash it for about a month. When I did wash it, I noticed gobs of hair coming out in the comb. When I washed my hair two weeks later, the same thing happened. I'm terrified."

In most cases, this hair loss is only temporary. Normal growth usually resumes about six months after you've had your baby. But it could take as long as a year for everything to return to the way it was before you were pregnant.

Hormones are also affected by your diet. If you overeat, binge diet, going from one extreme diet to another, or suffer from anorexia nervosa, you upset your hormonal balance and slow the growth rate of hair.

Similarly, if you've been nervous, upset, anxious, or sick with a serious illness, your hair may thin. Mental and physical stresses are big factors. During periods of acute stress, your hormone levels bounce around and you may lose patches of hair or have thinning. But if you seek the proper treatment for the stress-related problem and recover, your hair is likely to grow back.

Sudden hair loss may signal that you have an immune system disorder. And because medical conditions are a distinct possibility, it is a good idea to see a dermatologist or your family physician, who can conduct blood tests to determine the problem.

Lupus, thyroid disease, and anemia are among the conditions that can be responsible for hair loss. Treating an underlying medical condition is very important for your overall well-being and can also help to promote normal hair growth.

Cancer patients who undergo chemotherapy treatments also experience hair loss. Usually the hair will grow back. You may see regrowth in two months, or it could take as long as a year. Dr. Downie says, "We often find that when the hair grows back after chemotherapy, it is not as thick as it once was."

Hair Care

If you are otherwise healthy and are torturing your hair, and most of us do, you're likely to have a problem. Coloring, perming, straightening, adding chemicals to your hair, and applying heat via a blow-dryer or curling iron damages the hair. What Jackie describes in her e-mail is typical: "I have several bald spots on my scalp as well as a burn from a perm. My hair is breaking off and it has gotten very thin in the past few years."

Certain hairstyles can also cause damage. Consistently pulling your hair back tightly puts traction on the roots, causing men and women to lose hair.

This is a particular problem for Sikh men who pull their long hair back in a tight bun. Japanese women who wear traditional hairstyles also have this kind of hair loss, as do African-Americans and Caribbean-Americans who are tightly braiding or twisting their hair and using extensions.

People with tightly coiled hair frequently tug harder at their hair than other people because of the construction of the hair itself. Tightly coiled hair curves as it comes out of the scalp. It requires more pressure to comb and to brush, and that force often causes damage that breaks the hair. The curve also prevents the scalp's natural oils from moving down individual hair shafts as it does in straight or wavy hair. Consequently, the hair is very dry. The drier and more brittle the hair, the greater the potential for breakage.

So tightly coiled hair is more vulnerable to damage than straight and wavy hair. The damage often starts when we style children's hair.

When parents begin tightly braiding their children's hair, or pulling it back in tight ponytails, the damage—known medically as *traction alopecia*—begins. As the children grow, the hair loss starts at the hairline and around the ears. There is also likely to be thinning at the forehead and at the back of the neck. Sometimes the damage is irreversible.

Dr. Cook-Bolden found, "As a mother I was so paranoid that I tried all sorts of nonpulling techniques on my daughter's hair. I made little curls with my fingers. I put it up in very loose ponytails, and sometimes I would give her a little French roll."

Fortunately, Dr. Cook-Bolden's daughter didn't like a hot comb applied to her hair. Many people use grease and hair oils to make the hair more flexible. Then they use a hot comb or iron to style it. The grease and the hot instruments often burn the scalp. Once you damage the scalp, there's a good chance that the hair won't grow back in that spot.

Because we are all caught up in the importance of our image, it is very difficult to give up the things that we think improve our appearance. But if you are worried about hair loss, it may be a good time to reconsider some of the things that you are doing and work on a new hair management plan.

What You Can Do on Your Own

The first thing that you want to do for yourself or your child is to make sure that you eliminate stress on the hair. Try to create hairstyles that are gentle and don't tug at the roots.

Children's Hair

When you style your child's hair, try making the ponytails a little looser. If you braid, make the braids a little looser. We know that you want your child to look good, and it is difficult to balance children's demands for the style of the moment with their long-term health and cosmetic needs.

In the course of a lifetime, depending on the texture of your child's hair, he or she may have plenty of chemical hair treatments. So try to put off perming for as long as you can. Those so-called kiddie perms with calcium hydroxide are not necessarily gentle enough. They can severely dry the hair. If you do perm, try to limit the amount of time the solution is on the head. Go for a slightly less relaxed look. Leave a little curl in the hair. The curlier the hairstyle and the less heat you apply, the healthier the hair will be in the long run.

Everyone's hair should be washed and conditioned at least once a week.

Adult Hair

The same cautions apply to adults.

If you or a stylist braid, twist, or put your hair up in any way, make sure it's not too tight and that bobby pins don't dig into your scalp. Nothing should hurt. Your brain shouldn't feel as if it is popping out of your scalp. We've seen many women with big scars in the center of their scalps and infections caused by hairdressers who gouged a piece out of them.

Men who braid their hair and put it up in tight styles should also be aware of the danger.

When you have a weave, ask the stylist *not* to use glue. When the weave is removed, you won't be able to separate your own hair from the glue, frequently causing the hair to come out in big chunks. The glue can also damage the scalp and create bald spots.

Dr. Downie says, "Riva wore weaves glued to her scalp for years. When she came to see me, she complained of hair loss and said her scalp never felt clean. In fact, fungus was growing under the glued weave, and it had penetrated her scalp and was permanently damaging the roots of her hair."

Relaxers and Chemical Treatments

Many men and women use perms, straighteners, or relaxers as part of their regular routine. We don't suggest that you apply any of these products by yourself. Dr. Downie has her hair relaxed once every six to eight weeks. She says, "I feel really strongly that any chemical process should be done by a professional. The risk of damage is too great for you to do this on your own at home."

There are two basic types of relaxers. Sodium hydroxide alkali relaxers are thick creams with a high acid content. If this is what your hairdresser uses, make sure that a petrolatum (petroleum jelly) product is used on your scalp to protect it. The very high acid level can cause the hair to swell and break. That's why a neutralization shampoo immediately follows the relaxer. The formula helps to restore the hair's acid, or pH, level.

> IMPORTANT: *Any chemical process should be done by a professional. The risk of damage is too great for you to do this on your own at home.*

Guanidine hydroxides formed with calcium are usually called the "no-lye" relaxers. But these relaxers can be more damaging than the sodium hydroxide type because people tend to leave them on longer. They take a long time to work, and the extra time on your scalp can harm and dry the hair. You may be better off using the sodium hydroxide relaxer.

Applying the relaxer correctly is important. Santa Cruz of the Santa Cruz Salon in New York City says the technique is the key to saving the hair from damage: "You should try to avoid putting the relaxer on the scalp. But you want to make sure that the relaxer is close to where the growth begins and doesn't overlap on to the already relaxed hair. There's likely to be a little leakage to the scalp. So it's important to pay attention. You want to apply the relaxer quickly and wash it off in six to eighteen minutes depending on the thickness of the hair." Immediately after the hair is relaxed and the solution is washed out with a shampoo designed for damaged hair, a moisturizing conditioner must be applied.

Color

New York stylist Dale Edgehill says, "Never color your hair on the same day you perm or relax. You must wait at least two weeks between each chemical process to avoid breaking or damaging your hair. African-Americans should never use bleach. After any color is applied, it's essential to wash with a shampoo for color-treated hair and the same type of moisturizing conditioner."

The Right Shampoo

All shampoos are not the same. There is a right kind of shampoo for chemically treated hair and a wrong kind. The shampoo you use can help to prevent breakage. When you have treated hair, you need to use a shampoo that is acid, or pH, balanced. Most shampoos contain alkaline, which can swell the hair shaft. The swelling can break relaxed, color-treated, and permed hair. Similarly the conditioner should contain an ingredient that is gentle and moisturizing and helps to balance the acid in your hair without breaking it.

If you have straight hair and are perming it to add body, curl, or waves, the same rules apply. Remove the harsh chemicals quickly from your hair, and use a conditioner after the shampoo.

Your regular hair management routine should also include a sensible hair washing schedule. Very dry hair can be washed once a week, and oily and normal hair may need to be washed more frequently.

Tara e-mailed us with a question we hear frequently: "I work out four to five times a week and I work up a pretty good sweat. My hair has a relaxer in it, and when it gets wet, it is hard to manage. How often should I wash it?"

This is a tough one. It is frustrating to try to wash your hair frequently when it is styled, but tightly coiled hair should be washed as soon as possible after working out if you sweat or after you swim. Sweat, chlorine, and saltwater make the hair porous and can cause it to break. Dr. Downie runs or works out about four times a week. She says, "I wash my hair once a week, if I'm not too sweaty. During the summer months I wash it two to three times a week, and I always wash it after I swim. This means I have to put moisture back into the hair through deep conditioners. After washing, I condition it with Aveda, Nioxin, or KeraCare products."

New York stylist Diane DaCosta says, "Tightly coiled hair requires a lot of moisture. Steam conditioners every two weeks can help to put moisture into the hair shaft."

When you blow-dry your hair or use a hot comb, try not to pull the hair too much. Be a little kinder to your hair and scalp. If your hairdresser is too rough, ask her to lighten up.

If you have tightly coiled or dry hair, Diane DaCosta recommends massaging your scalp with an essential oil every day. "It is especially important when you have weaves, braids, locks, or twists, because you're not manipulating the hair on a daily basis," she says. Diane recommends almond oil for moisturizing, lavender for conditioning, rosemary for stimulating the scalp, and sage and chamomile for calming treatments.

But beware. Many people are allergic to both natural and synthetic botanicals. Before you put anything on your hair or scalp, test a very small amount in the crook of your arm. Wait a week to see if there is a reaction. If you don't have a reaction, then enjoy using the botanicals.

A number of companies specialize in shampoos and conditioners for damaged hair. Many stylists recommend Matrix shampoos and conditioners for curly, dry, and flyaway hair. These products seem to help keep the hair sleek and straight. Aveda has a line of botanical products called Curessence that contains proteins and glycerin from Brazil nuts. Avlon has the KeraCare line of products, and Nexus has a range of shampoos and conditioners that work well for all hair types. All of these products can be purchased in drugstores, beauty supply shops, and salons and via the Internet. Essential oils can be purchased for between $5 and $10 a bottle in herbal shops such as Aphrodisia in New York City.

Blow-Drying

For those of us who depend on this technique, it is a necessary evil. Heat can easily damage and break all types of hair.

Television hairstylist Diane D'Agostino says the method and tools you use can reduce damage and add shine. She says, "Try using a diffuser on the end of the dryer to soften the heat and reduce the chance of damaging the hair." The right brush is important. Diane recommends a Mason Pearson brush with natural or mixed bristles. The flat brush helps spread the natural oils down the hair shaft. She says, "When you are finished blowing, the hair will have a nice healthy look. Before you begin to blow-dry, section off the hair with clips. Blow one section at a time. Hold the brush at the root and move it away from the scalp toward the tip of the hair following with heat. Hold the dryer a few inches away from the hair. It's important to be patient and not to tug at the hair."

Dandruff

Blow-drying and other styling techniques can cause dandruff. Dandruff is a very common problem, and it is troublesome particularly for people with tightly coiled hair who tend to have dry scalps and dry hair. The lack of oil on the scalp and the hair shaft causes the flaky dandruff. Dr. Downie says, "Black women seem to suffer disproportionately from dandruff. Infrequent washing and the buildup of products on the scalp may aggravate the condition."

People with all hair types may experience dandruff when the seasons change and the air becomes colder and drier. Hormonal changes, stress, and scratching the scalp may also cause dandruff.

It is possible for dandruff to spread from the scalp to the neck and ears. Some people develop dandruff in their eyebrows, eyelashes, beard, or mustache.

Dandruff can be controlled. But it is important to treat it as soon as it appears. There are excellent over-the-counter shampoos. We recommend Nizoral AD shampoo and Neutrogena T Gel. If the dandruff persists, you may want to see a dermatologist, who is likely to prescribe a stronger shampoo, such as Nizoral 2%, Loprox, or Capex.

> TIP: *If you have dandruff, it is a good idea to shampoo every day and to massage a heavy lather into your scalp. Make sure that you rinse thoroughly and remove all of the shampoo from your hair and scalp.*

These shampoos can also be used to help control dandruff that has spread to your ears, neck, or face. Gentle baby shampoos can also help reduce the dandruff around the eyes.

If you have dandruff, it is a good idea to shampoo every day and to massage a heavy lather into your scalp. Make sure that you rinse thoroughly and remove all of the shampoo from your hair and scalp.

A Doctor's Guidance

Regardless of what you do to improve your hair care, it is possible that your problems will persist. A knowledgeable doctor can help you reverse some of the damage to your hair and scalp.

Styling damage often causes swelling around the root of the hair. If that's the case, the doctor will likely use a combination of therapies including anti-inflammatory injections to the scalp to calm the swelling and inflammation. The doctor may also prescribe topical creams, gels, or solutions. The treatment depends on the severity of your problem and what can be accomplished realistically.

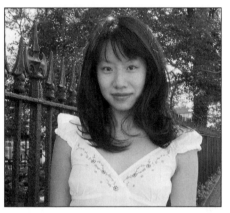

As the scalp inflammation eases, the doctor may recommend either 2 percent or 5 percent Rogaine solution, which can be purchased over the counter. Rogaine works for about 50 percent of the people who use it, but it is possible that it may irritate your scalp.

If you decide to use it, apply it carefully with the dropper included in the package. When it works, Rogaine produces hair growth wherever it is applied, and you may end up with hair in unwanted places. To prevent unwanted growth, Dr. Cook-Bolden prescribes Vaniqa, a cream that blocks the hair growth enzyme. You can apply the Vaniqa to your forehead and cheeks at the same time you use Rogaine around your hairline.

Rogaine will cost about $40 a month. If you try the treatments twice a day for six months to a year and you're not satisfied, you may want to consider hair transplants. They are expensive, but they can be effective. Hair transplants generally cost between $4,000 and $15,000.

The Bottom Line

The statistics are in our genes. Many of us will lose some or even all of our hair naturally and yet others will inadvertently create hair loss with hair styling. You can reverse the trend by discovering the ways to treat your hair *gently*.

Hairline
Neck
Bumps

CHAPTER 18

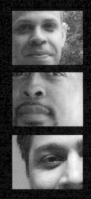

IRRITATED RAISED BUMPS ON THE BACK OF THE NECK FALL INTO THE category of small but incredibly annoying things that appear primarily in skin of color.

Actually, it's a medical condition called *acne keloidalis nuchae.* Doctors have known about this problem for hundreds of years, but that doesn't soothe men like Rasheed, who wrote asking for help: "I started to discover bumps at the bottom of my neck about a year ago. The bumps are not only eyesores, they are also very itchy and generally uncomfortable. The bumps have spread to virtually all of my scalp and they continue to bleed. Please help me fix this."

Rasheed has a particularly bad case of hairline bumps. It is not unusual for them to appear on the scalp as well. Although you can do a few simple things right away, you may need the help of a doctor.

Why It Happens

We can treat the bumps, even though we're not really sure what causes them. One of the most obvious theories centers on how your hair is cut and your neck is shaved. We notice that bumps appear after a short haircut is given. Many people have their necks or hairlines shaved with a razor to create a neat appearance. That's a problem. Two things can happen. Very often a razor nicks the skin and scar tissue grows, covering the nick and creating a hairline neck bump. Or, when a razor cuts individual curly hairs, it leaves sharp ends on the hair. Those sharp ends often curl back into the skin, creating razor bumps (see page 138 for more on this).

This happens most frequently to African-American, Caribbean, Latino, and Asian men. Women get the bumps, too, but it seems to be a bigger problem with men. Typically we hear from men like Alex, who says, "I have numerous bumps growing on the back of my head. They started to appear after I had my head shaved." That's not surprising. Most barbers follow sanitary and safe procedures. But if the barber does nick you, he should let you know right away so that you can treat the cut before it leads to problems.

Whether you shave your head or have a barber do it, the process can bring on the bumps. And if you have a condition like Alex describes, the bumps may merge together to form a thick scar.

Researchers also suggest a number of other causes. These causes may be complicated medical issues like an immune system disorder, an increase of skin cells at the particular spot, bacterial infections, and infections caused by dirty hair clippers. A commonsense explanation involves your clothes. Your shirt collars may irritate the skin at the neckline and make the climate ripe for the bumps.

Remedies
What You Can Do on Your Own

You can start to help yourself before you even get a bump. Changing a few basic habits is the best approach. When you get a haircut, avoid having the neck or the back of the head trimmed too closely with a razor. You want to be certain that your barber uses sterile equipment and is careful about his work. He should cut the hair without cutting the skin. You might consider asking the barber to trim the hair at the neckline with a sharp scissors rather than a razor.

Because your clothing may irritate your skin, try to eliminate anything from your wardrobe that is tight fitting or rubs the back of your neck. Harsh clothing detergents may aggravate the condition. You can minimize irritation by using fragrance-free detergents such as All Free or Cheer Free when you wash your clothes.

When a bump appears, no amount of scrubbing or picking will make it go away. Any aggressive and abrasive action is likely only to continue to inflame the bumps and cause infection. It's like waving the red shirt at the bull. The bump probably will get bigger and even more uncomfortable. It's really important to make sure that the bumps don't become infected.

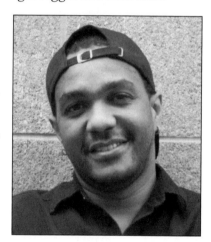

At-home remedies are usually temporary stopgaps. This is really one of those skin management issues that requires the attention of a doctor. If you're serious about tackling the problem, it's a good idea to seek the advice of a dermatologist who can help to get the bumps under control.

A Doctor's Guidance

For this medical condition, we've found that combination therapy works best. And because the bumps aren't the same on everyone's skin, doctors vary the treatment depending on the individual. A doctor may prescribe a retinoid, like Retin-A Micro, to be applied to the bumps at night. It contains a derivative of vitamin A that speeds the natural shedding of dead skin and makes the new skin smoother and healthier. A topical steroid applied to the area can help to decrease the inflammation and irritation. A doctor may also recommend a topical or oral antibiotic to calm any infection and inflammation.

If the bumps become very inflamed a doctor may inject them with a low potency steroid to flatten them and decrease the inflammation. You're likely to need a series of shots at least twice a month for several months.

We see the best response and the quickest healing in patients who seek treatment early. It is possible, however, that the bumps won't respond and you may require surgery.

Doctors regularly flatten neck bumps with a laser. It is important that the doctor use a laser that will not harm the pigment cells in skin of color. Laser treatment is likely to remove the hair in that area, which is something you may want to consider. But laser treatments can be very effective.

If the hairline bumps have merged into one mass, producing a thick shiny scar, the doctor may remove the mass with a conventional surgical scalpel. Often the doctor will cut deep into the layers of the skin to reach the bottom of the bump. If the bump is removed, the wound is likely to be very tender and could take as long as twelve weeks to heal. It is also possible that the doctor will stitch the area after the scar has been removed. It's important for the doctor to monitor the healing process. During postsurgery follow-up visits, the doctor is likely to inject a steroid twice a month for at least six months to prevent the bumps from reappearing. It's not a quick process but the results can be significant.

Dr. Cook-Bolden says, "Laser treatments before and after surgery can help to prevent the mass from growing back."

The Bottom Line

Hairline neck bumps can be managed, brought under control, and even eliminated. Because a combination of therapies may be required, you'll have to follow through on the treatments and follow the doctor's directions carefully.

Hair
Removal
CHAPTER 19

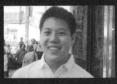

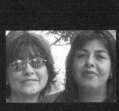

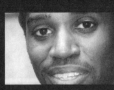

WE'VE BEEN TRYING TO GET RID OF UNWANTED HAIR FOR CENTURIES. Twenty thousand years ago, our dark-skinned ancestors drew pictures of their daily rituals on cave walls depicting themselves shaving with sharpened rocks and shells.

We've evolved some since then. The advent of the laser, and the refinement that has made the laser safe for dark skin, have opened up new possibilities. Dr. Cook-Bolden says, "Using these lasers has revolutionized the way we can treat both men and women with olive and dark skin. And it has really made it so much easier for people of color who have problems with facial hair, or who simply want to remove hair from other parts of their bodies."

But many of us still use daily hair removal methods that are pretty close to primitive.

Whether you are man who regularly shaves his beard, or a woman who removes hair from her face, her legs, or bikini area, you know that the hair removal process is time consuming, often painful, and can damage and discolor your skin.

Increasingly, people are considering hair removal in what were once considered unusual places. Men regularly have hair removed from their necks and their backs. Some people want hair removed from their entire body, and that's possible. But all hair removal on skin of color must be conducted with great care.

Dr. Downie says, "I've seen terrible burns in the most sensitive areas, like the groin, from improper waxing. The wax was simply too hot. Sheila came to me after she'd been burned and developed large keloids, very thick scars, in her groin and on her inner thighs. Now she can't even wear a normal bathing suit."

And that's exactly what happened to Jasmine, who wrote to us asking for help: "I'm embarrassed to wear a bathing suit. I have very dark discoloration and scars. This happened because of waxing."

We've talked about it earlier, but it is worth repeating: if you have any color in your skin, the melanocytes—cells that give the skin pigment—are especially active. Any kind of irritation, or trauma, can make the melanocytes more active, and they produce more color.

Some people think that because they have a lighter complexion this may not be a problem for them. Dr. Cook-Bolden says, "Patients of Asian and Latino descent whose skin tone is very fair can have very sensitive skin and unstable pigment cells. The same precautions should be taken when treating *all* patients of color."

Remedies

What You Can Do on Your Own

A variety of hair removal methods exist, which you may know quite well. But we may be able to give you a few tips in this review. We've already described the most effective shaving methods in chapter 15 on male facial hair. So we'll start with depilatories, which many people use at home.

Depilatories

You may have just discovered depilatories in the drugstore, but they've been used for centuries. Researchers think that women in 4000 B.C. made a paste of natural arsenic, quicklime, and starch to remove their hair. The concoction worked the same way as modern depilatories; chemicals dissolve hair, but leave the roots in place.

Although modern formulas are more sophisticated, ingredients in depilatories can still be harsh and irritating. Some depilatories contain sulfur. And they smell. Others contain perfumes and are especially irritating. Remember, your skin is already sensitive.

This is not our favorite method of hair removal, but we understand that depilatories are relatively inexpensive and popular. People like them because they can remove the hair for four days to a week. If you do use one, make sure that you follow the instructions. If we had to pick a product, we'd choose Nair. But make sure that you buy the appropriate product. There's Nair for the body, and there's a gentler Nair for the face. People whose skin can tolerate it find that Nair does the job. Test it first on a small area on your arm or leg before applying it. If you use a depilatory, minimize the irritation by applying and removing the depilatory quickly.

Egyptian Hair Threading

You can tell by the name. It's believed that hair threading began in ancient Egypt. Women in the Middle East, India, Turkey, Africa, and Asia regularly use Egyptian hair threading to remove hair. And while you can't remove the hair with one sweep as you can with a depilatory, Dr. Cook-Bolden describes this as "a very gentle form of tweezing." But she, along with many other women, find it difficult to locate a knowledgeable threader.

Although the process is simple, it requires skill. The threader twists a cotton thread along a row of hair and pulls the hair out. The roots of the hairs are not destroyed and that means the hair will grow back. Hair could grow back after a week or after three to four weeks depending on the pattern of your hair growth.

Electrolysis

Electrolysis, on the other hand, is a process that may permanently remove some hair. But it requires patience, time, and money. And if needles upset you, this method is not for you. Dr. Downie tried it. She was eager to remove three stubborn chin hairs. The electrologist removed two, and Dr. Downie wouldn't let her do the third. "It was too painful. I made her stop."

But electrolysis is effective because it destroys the hair at the root. However, it can take you a lifetime to remove all of the hair on your face. It is a slow, long-term effort targeting one hair at a time.

During short sessions, an aesthetician inserts a needle, connected to an electronic device, into a hair follicle. A quick surge of electrical current zaps the root of the hair and prevents it from growing back. Though it is effective, many people find it painful and limit the sessions to between five and thirty minutes.

Even if you could endure hours and hours of electrolysis in one sitting, it wouldn't remove all of the hair. Hair grows in cycles. Every hair doesn't pop out at the same time. Hairs in the dermal layer of the skin are always working their way to the surface. That's why multiple treatments are required.

Aestheticians must have special certifications and licenses to practice electrolysis. Do not let anyone use this technique on you unless you see the certification and the license.

COST

The price of electrolysis will vary. Usually an electrologist charges for the amount of time the procedure takes. The price may range from $20 to $120 or more.

Waxing

Waxing is a tried and true method for many of us. With waxing you may be hair-free for two to six weeks depending on your hair growth.

Whether you're having a facial wax on the beard area, the upper lip, or the eyebrows; a conventional bikini wax; or an all-the-way Brazilian, waxing should be done properly to avoid irritation and the possibility of ingrown hairs.

You can take a few steps to minimize problems. You want to make sure that the skin isn't already sensitive. So if you use any retinoids like Retin-A Micro, Renova, or fading creams, you should stop three to five days before you wax.

Over-the-counter alpha and beta hydroxy products aren't as strong as prescription preparations or the products that doctors use. But if you are using them in the area that you'd like to wax, you may want to take a break from those products for a few days before the wax.

Your eyebrow area is not exempt from this rule. Even if you think you are not using the retinoid or the fade cream near your eyebrows, these products leave a lingering effect.

"I've seen the skin pulled off around the eyebrow and the upper lip because a woman used a retinoid before she went to have her eyebrows and lip waxed," Dr. Cook-Bolden says. "We can help it to heal, but it is a serious problem."

Many salons want to get you in and out quickly, and frequently the waxer will neglect to test the temperature of the wax. We've seen too many women badly burned. And those burns turn to dark scars.

You want to make sure that your skin is free of moisturizer and perfectly clean before it is waxed. Jin Soon Choi, of Jin Soon Natural Hand and Foot Spas in New York City, will apply a fine layer of baby powder to the skin before she applies the wax. "This gives extra protection to the skin," she says.

A cold wax is the preferred method for people with sensitive skin. At the Yana Herbal Beauty Salon in New York City, Yana Yusupidi and her daughter Helena Narimanidze regularly use a cold wax on their clients, including actresses Sarah Jessica Parker and Marisa Tomei. Yana makes her own cold wax with lemon juice, sugar, and honey in a formula created by her grandmother in their native Georgia, which was once part of the former Soviet Union.

When it's applied, a ball of cold wax is rolled over the hairy area. The hair clings to the sugary substance and is removed almost painlessly. Yana says, "In Georgia, honey has been used for centuries to heal skin irritations. The advantage of this cold wax is that it doesn't irritate the veins, capillaries, or the most sensitive skin."

Cold waxes are available in many salons in different formulations. Most salons routinely use warm wax, which should be just a little warmer than body temperature when applied to the skin. Dr. Downie suggests asking the waxer to test the temperature on her gloved hand or wrist. When an aesthetician applies wax and then uses a cloth strip to remove it, it is important to make sure that all of the hair adheres to the cloth on the first pull. Repeatedly applying wax and then pulling at the same area can damage the skin. The strip should be pulled back at an angle so that the hair is removed at the root and the skin isn't bruised. At the Elizabeth Arden Salon, aesthetician Diane Greene says, "We are very careful with skin of color. We apply a thick coating of our patented organic beeswax directly onto the skin using a metal spatula or spoon. The wax hardens in seconds and we remove the hair by pulling the wax in the opposite direction from which the hair grows. We've found that this method is the most effective and least likely to damage the skin."

After the wax, the skin should be cleaned with a mild cleanser and warm water followed by the application of a soothing moisturizer. Many waxers stock products that are spiked with natural botanicals including aloe vera, which may irritate your skin. Ask the waxer to tell you what she uses before she applies it. Sometimes unscented baby oil is the best lubricant to remove the wax and soothe the skin.

Waxing makes the skin tender. Even though you've got a clean, sleek look, avoid going out into the sun immediately. The sun will stimulate the skin pigment cells that have already been stirred up by the action of the waxing and you can end up with dark marks.

If the waxed areas are going to be exposed to the sun, you need sun protection. We like sun protection with Parsol 1789, UVA and UVB protection, zinc oxide or titanium dioxide, and a sun protection factor of 30.

It is possible that even if the waxer does everything right, your skin will be irritated. If it is, your dermatologist may prescribe an anti-inflammatory cream to decrease the irritation.

A Doctor's Guidance

A dermatologist can help you tackle your hair removal problems in a more scientific way. The simplest solution is Vaniqa, a relatively new prescription medicine which Dr. Cook-Bolden likes very much. It doesn't remove the hair, but it reduces it. "My patients like it because it slows down the hair growth," she says.

Vaniqa is a cream that blocks the enzyme that causes hair to grow. It's slightly labor intensive. You have to apply it to your skin twice a day. But before you begin to use it, we recommend that you patch-test Vaniqa on a small area of your skin. You want to make sure that it doesn't irritate. Vaniqa also requires patience. It takes at least eight weeks to achieve the best results.

If your hair growth is thick, it may be necessary to use Vaniqa in conjunction with other hair removal methods. "Even if people decide that they want to continue to shave, they find that they have to shave less often when they use Vaniqa," Dr. Cook-Bolden says.

She also prescribes Vaniqa when patients undergo laser hair

removal treatments, although she advises them to stop using the medication five days before the laser treatments.

Laser Hair Removal

In a 2001 study, Dr. Cook-Bolden concluded that laser treatments are effective in skin of color for hair removal and the treatment of razor bumps. The study found that the laser removed the hair without irritating the skin and further aggravating the bumps. And when the hair was removed, the razor bumps didn't form. Dr. Cook-Bolden also confirmed what other researchers previously discovered when studying the laser's effect on lighter skin. In dark skin and light skin, the laser can stimulate the body's natural collagen. Since collagen gives the skin texture and resilience, the laser can, in many cases, improve the quality of the skin.

It is only relatively recently that the laser has been found safe for dark skin. Although dermatologists have been practicing laser hair removal since the early 1990s, the lasers they used initially could damage dark skin.

To make sense of all this, it may help to understand how the laser works. The word *laser* stands for *l*ight *a*mplification by *s*timulated *e*mission of *r*adiation. That means the laser creates energy in the form of a coherent beam of light, which is used in many different ways in medicine and technology.

Lasers harness specific colors of light and produce different amounts of heat or energy directed in a very narrow focus. The laser's energy can pass through the outer layers of the skin and target the hair follicles. The color in the hair follicle absorbs the laser heat and the follicle is destroyed. That's how it works, ideally.

But early lasers damaged skin of color. The energy was absorbed by the dark melanin, or pigment, in skin of color in the same way that the pigment in the hair follicle absorbed the energy. People of color who had this procedure were burned and often lost pigment in their skin.

Recently new lasers were introduced and approved by the FDA. These lasers have longer wavelengths. They can be set to direct the light through the skin to attack the hair follicle without harming the skin. This was a major advance and an important step for treating skin of color.

We want to warn you. There are people performing laser procedures who should not be doing this kind of work.

If you are having laser hair removal, we recommend that you choose a board-certified dermatologist or plastic surgeon who is properly trained and has the correct equipment. There is serious concern about scarring, burns, and permanent skin discoloration after laser procedures performed by people who aren't qualified. The American Society for Dermatologic Surgery reports an alarming increase in the number of patients who have sought out remedial treatment after being hurt by untrained doctors and nonphysicians performing laser procedures.

When you choose the right doctor, it is important that the doctor test areas of your skin to find the correct setting. Everyone's skin reacts differently and your doctor must understand that. The doctor may do several tests before committing to do the laser hair removal.

Typically a doctor will apply a cooling gel to the area before treating you. It's possible that a local anesthetic may also be used. The sensation of laser hair removal feels like a rubber band snap. There is a slight tingling. The amount of pain you experience depends on the type of laser being used.

The doctor directs the laser's energy to the specific target area and then moves on to an adjacent area. The procedure is quick. The treatments last anywhere from five to twenty minutes depending on the area being treated; it is more time consuming to treat a larger area such as the legs. Don't be disappointed if you don't have instant results. It takes awhile to see the outcome. And depending on your hair growth and what you want to achieve, you may need three to five treatments before you notice a difference.

Laser hair removal is effective for facial hair, and it is particularly good for men who want to remove hair in strategic areas where they've been having problems with razor bumps. The doctor can target the neck and cheeks where the razor bumps flare up, but leave hair in the mustache area and on the chin.

The laser can also be used to remove hair anywhere on the body, and it's becoming increasingly popular with both women and men.

Walter went to see Dr. Downie because his back was very hairy. He wanted to remove the hair before his wedding day. "I treated him with a Lyra Nd:Yag laser once a month for six months and we were able to remove all of the hair," Dr. Downie says.

The laser will remove the hair for one to three months. When the hair grows back, it is likely to be thinner. It may permanently remove some hairs, but that is not always the case. Laser hair removal is *not* permanent. The FDA allows people to advertise that hair removal is permanent if it takes longer than two months to grow back. But to us, two months isn't permanent.

COST

The price of laser hair removal will vary depending on the skill of the physician and where you live. It is likely to cost at least $400 a session. Many doctors will create a package price for a number of treatments and that could reduce the cost. But a series of treatments over a year or more may cost as much as $5,000.

Intense Pulsed Light

Intense pulsed light treatment is a nonlaser procedure that has also been found to remove hair safely and effectively. Whereas the laser uses a single, or coherent beam of light, IPL technology uses many beams of light. Bursts of light penetrate the skin to target and remove hairs. The treatment is performed in a doctor's office with a wandlike instrument that is part of a computer-generated system that produces and controls the light. During the treatment you may feel as though you're being zapped by a rubber band. Treatments last from five to fifteen minutes, and there may be some redness or swelling, which should disappear in a few hours.

You are likely to require three or four treatments over the course of several months. This is not a permanent hair removal method, although some people report that their hair growth is significantly reduced after repeated treatments.

COST

The price of IPL treatments is likely to vary. A single session may cost $400, and doctors are likely to arrange package prices for multiple sessions.

The Bottom Line

Whether you are waxing, using an Egyptian threader, an aesthetician who is licensed to practice electrolysis, or a doctor to perform laser hair removal or intense pulsed light treatments, it is important to choose that professional carefully. Not everyone is familiar with skin of color. And although you want to remove the hair, you don't want to permanently darken or damage your skin.

Joint
Darkness
CHAPTER 20

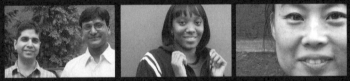

Elbows, Knees, Fingers, and Toes

If you've been secretly staring at your joints trying to figure out why the skin there is darker than the rest of you, don't worry. You are in good company. Skin of color ranging from the palest Asian tone to olive and the darkest of dark skin is prone to darkening in certain areas. But people are often too embarrassed to talk about it.

Lala writes: "I feel silly. I'm a twenty-eight-year-old Asian woman and maybe I should be worrying about other things. But it's embarrassing. My knees and elbows are darker than the rest of my skin and so are my toes. My toes are the worst. I hate to wear sandals because I'm afraid people will stare."

It's a shame to feel that you have to hide your toes. Yet it is not unusual for people to have severe discoloration that they want to cover up.

That's what Tanika says she does: "I have a light-brown complexion. But my joints and elbows are black. It's been like this since I was a little girl, and I'm twenty-two years old now. Since I started to work I've never worn skirts, and I always wear long sleeves. I've tried using creams from the drugstore and they don't work. Is there anything that I can do?"

Over-the-counter creams and lotions aren't likely to work if the problem is severe or genetic. But in many cases there is a combination of things that you can do.

Why It Happens

Some people are born with darker skin on their joints. If this is a genetic problem, it may be impossible to make a significant difference.

For many others, the darkness is caused by friction and the way your skin has responded to it.

If you're like the rest of us, you started banging your elbows and knees when you were very young. We crawl. We fall. We put our elbows on the table. We're rough with our fingers and toes. We jam our feet into shoes that are too tight. These are natural actions that result in tiny traumas to the skin. We're all born with extra skin at the joints so that we can bend and stretch. If you have skin of color, that extra skin darkens easily.

> FACT: *Some people are born with darker skin on their joints. If this is a genetic problem, it may be impossible to make a significant difference.*
>
> *For many others, the darkness is caused by friction and the way your skin has responded to it.*

Throughout this book, we describe what makes dark skin special, and it is worth restating: the melanocytes, the cells that give our skin color, are very active in Asian, olive, and dark skin. The slightest bump, bruise, scrape, or trauma of any kind gets those melanocytes working overtime. They become extremely active. In the joint areas, the extra color cells get trapped in the extra skin. So if you are doing housework, or anything that involves repeated pressure on your knees and elbows for long periods of time, it's likely that the skin over those joints will darken. Similarly, if you are doing a type of work or playing a game or sport that is rough on your hands, your knuckles are likely to be darker than the rest of your skin. The same is true for your toes. If you squeeze your feet into great-looking shoes that hurt, and your toes get scrunched up, your toe joints are likely to be darker than the rest of the skin.

Even if you've built up the dark spots over years of tiny abuses, you can begin to make an improvement now.

Remedies

What You Can Do on Your Own

First, don't try to rub away the darkness. It won't work.

Violet used Ajax, Clorox, and a pumice stone to try to erase the dark marks on her toe joints. Instead she scrubbed her skin raw and stripped the pigment from the skin on her toe joints. She panicked and went to see Dr. Downie. "As soon as I learned what she was doing to herself, I advised her to stop. We're working to even the pigment with chemical peels that will speed the restoration of new skin cells. But you can't always correct the problem once the damage has been done," Dr. Downie says.

In all situations, it's really important to treat your skin *gently*.

Think about your habits and the way your body moves and works. If you can eliminate some of the damaging action, you'll stop creating new dark skin cells, which will be a big step forward.

Sunblock may not sound like an immediately obvious solution, but it is very important. Once the skin gets dark in an area, the dark areas of the skin and the sun attract each other. It doesn't matter how dark you are or how dark your dark areas are; the sun will make them darker. At the risk of repeating ourselves, we recommend a sunblock with UVA and UVB, Parsol 1789, and a sun protection factor of at least 20. Apply the sunblock on every area exposed to the sun, paying particular attention to the joints.

Dr. Downie recommends that her patients use knee pads when they are playing contact sports, bathing their children, doing housework, or gardening. "It may sound extreme, but if people are banging their elbows around the computer, they should also wear elbow pads," she says.

Moisturizer is also important. Lubricate dry areas.

In chapter 2 on acne and chapter 7 on chemical peels, we describe the use of alpha hydroxy acids and retinoids. Products containing alpha hydroxy acids and retinoids are also important for treating darkened joints.

Because there is likely to be rough skin in these areas, it is a good idea to try to thin the skin a little bit with a lactic acid product. Moisturizers containing lactic acid include AmLactin, LactiCare, and

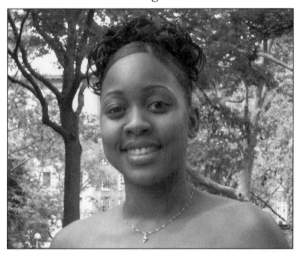

LAC-HYDRIN. They are available over the counter in most drugstores. Jergens Ash Relief is an excellent moisturizer containing beta hydroxy acid, and Eucerin Alpha Hydroxy Moisturizer is also a potent moisturizer.

As you are thinning the skin, you also want to begin to try to slough off the dead, dark skin cells and fade what's left behind. And that's where the vitamin A, or retinoid, products and other alpha and beta hydroxy acids come in. Over-the-counter products are a good way to begin to lighten the joints.

A Doctor's Guidance

A good doctor will immediately check to see if the problem is caused by a medical condition like psoriasis or keratoderma (see chapter 22). If it is, the dermatologist will treat that condition as she or he works to help you fade the darkness on the joints.

If there is not an underlying medical condition, a dermatologist will use a combination of therapies to even the skin tone. Many of the techniques that the dermatologist will use are described in chapter 12 on dark marks. But because the extra skin at the joints makes the darkness more difficult to treat than most other dark marks, the doctor may use stronger medications, including prescription moisturizers.

> FACT: *Because the extra skin at the joints makes the darkness more difficult to treat than most other dark marks, the doctor may use stronger medications, including prescription moisturizers.*

"When the dark areas are very resistant, I'll prescribe Carmol 40 or Vanamide, which contain urea. I may alternatively prescribe a specially compounded salicylic acid preparation. These can be very helpful," Dr. Cook-Bolden says.

A number of prescription medications work well together.

Hydroquinone, which blocks the enzyme that produces color in the melanocytes, serves to even out skin color. A doctor may prescribe at least a 4 percent hydroquinone product. It's most effective when combined with retinoids like Retin-A Micro. This is a full-strength retinoid that evens skin tone as it speeds the shedding of dead skin cells. It also stimulates natural collagen production and gives the skin a nice texture. Potent alpha and beta hydroxy acids can also be part of this equation. They speed up the exfoliation of dead skin cells and improve the collagen.

Some prescription medications contain all of these ingredients and others, including vitamins C and E, which are antioxidants that fight the oxygen compounds known as free radicals that cause aging. The combination prescription medications include EpiQuin Micro, Glyquin XM, and Alustra.

If the skin is very thick and very dark, the doctor may prescribe Tri-Luma Cream, another combination medication that contains a hydroquinone, a retinoid, and a steroid, as well as the other therapies. The medication should be used for a limited time and be monitored carefully by a doctor. Although a doctor may recommend Tri-Luma Cream for lightening joints, it has been approved by the FDA only for use in treating melasma. That means the company can advertise it only for that purpose. But doctors frequently find that medication approved by the FDA for one purpose is useful for treating other ailments as well.

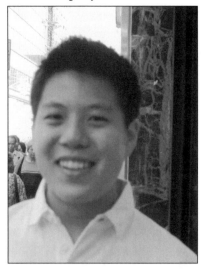

It is also possible that the doctor might prescribe a very potent retinoid like Tazorac, which has been effective on dark joints.

Microdermabrasion and a series of chemical peels performed over several months can speed the work of topical creams. Of the many chemical peels, beta hydroxy, or salicylic acid, peels may be the most effective.

The Bottom Line

Like so many other issues involving skin of color, there is no longer any need to struggle alone or be embarrassed about conditions that you share with billions of people all over the world. With proper attention and care, you can correct problems that arise because of the nature of your special skin.

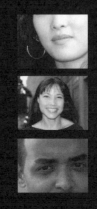

Keloids

CHAPTER 21

DEPENDING ON THE SEVERITY, WHEN MOST PEOPLE GET A CUT, A scrape, or a burn, it may leave a scar or a faint mark. And usually, even the most serious scars remain flat and may partially fade over time. But if you are prone to develop a keloid, you know the scar doesn't get better. It doesn't fade or go away. Keloid scars gets worse. They become hard and raised and often extend beyond the lines of the original scar.

The problem is that you won't learn whether your body forms keloids until the first one appears. When Faith was thirteen, she had her ears pierced: "The hole in my left ear didn't heal properly. This big, brown bump formed over the hole. No matter what I've tried, I've been unable to get rid of it. It is not only ugly, it's embarrassing. People stare at me all the time. When I was little, kids in school made fun of me. In cold weather, it hurts. And it itches most of the time. Is there anything that I can do?"

Keloids are a tough problem. And the truth is that treatment is not always effective. Keloids are still a medical mystery even though a scientist first described the thick raised scar in 1790, and it's suspected that people have dealt with keloids for thousands of years. There are accounts of early tribal and sexual rituals in which keloids were prized as marks of distinction.

Why It Happens

We'd like nothing better than to discover the cause of and a cure for keloids. This is another area involving skin of color that hasn't been researched extensively. Past attempts to study keloids have been frustrating. Funding to support research was limited because it was perceived as an ethnic medical issue with limited interest and appeal. That's changing. Scientists are once again trying to determine why keloids occur and how they can be prevented.

This is what we do know: keloids aren't cancers. And what happened to Faith is typical. Usually a keloid forms after a piercing, a sorority or fraternity branding, a cut, surgery, vaccinations, a bug or animal bite, tattooing, or anything else that disrupts the skin. As the skin heals, the cells multiply more than they should. During the healing process, if a body is prone to keloids, you will produce too many skin cells, which will build up over the injured area. In other words, there's excessive healing.

Researchers have found that excess collagen is produced as the wound heals. Collagen is the fiber that gives your skin elasticity and texture and helps plump up the skin. But in the case of a keloid, there is so much extra collagen that the scar heals with a thick raised coat.

To complicate the puzzle, some people develop keloids over areas of skin that don't appear to be damaged. You may have some irritation that you didn't notice. That's very common. Dr. Cook-Bolden's patient Alexandra developed five small keloids on her chest. She couldn't remember ever having an injury. Dr. Cook-Bolden discovered they were caused by a few acnelike bumps that had become inflamed and healed as keloids. "She was very upset because the keloids were disfiguring, and she had to wear turtlenecks and high-necked dresses all the time," Dr. Cook-Bolden says.

Keloids may be genetic, but there has been no scientific confirmation of this. And although people with light skin can develop keloids, they are much more likely to develop in people of African and Asian descent, as well as in the skin of people whose families are originally from the Indian subcontinent, Latin America, the Mediterranean, and the Middle East. We simply do not know why skin of color is more prone to developing keloids.

It may involve the protein structure of dark skin. The collagen fibers that give the skin structure are thicker in dark skin than they are in white skin, and the protein may cause the overhealing effect that produces too much scar tissue.

As Faith found out, keloids don't necessarily appear after the first nick or scrape of childhood. A child may experience all of the normal scrapes and bruises without developing a keloid until she or he is thirteen or fourteen years old. It's rare to develop a keloid before you reach adolescence. Keloids seem to appear in people who are between thirteen and forty years old, though the ages can vary. A baby who has her ears pierced before she's two years old may not have a problem. But when the same girl is fourteen and she puts another hole in her ear, she may then develop a keloid.

Remedies

What You Can Do on Your Own

Unfortunately, there isn't much you can do on your own besides treating your skin as *gently* as possible. If someone in your family has a keloid, then it is not a good idea for you to get a tattoo or a piercing. Any surgery poses a risk that the healing scar will form as a keloid. We've seen terrible keloids form after breast reductions, tummy tucks, liposuction, and some laser procedures. If there is even the remote possibility that you will develop a keloid, you're better off avoiding anything that traumatizes the skin. For mandatory surgery, it is important that you talk to your surgeon and detail your family history of keloid formation.

Because of the lack of definitive information, we know that those of you who suffer with keloids are eager for any information and any product that may help. Many so-called keloid remedies are widely advertised on the Internet, television, and the radio. It is all too easy to spend your money and pin your hopes on something that is not fully tested or proven to be effective.

Some manufacturers claim that their products will help. So-called keloid remedies include products with silicone sheeting. Although there is some evidence that silicone may be useful for treating nonkeloid scars, there isn't enough research to support the claims that silicone works for keloids.

Like other problems directly related to skin of color, you can manage a keloid with a qualified doctor's help.

A Doctor's Guidance

A dermatologist who is knowledgeable about treating skin of color won't make promises that she or he can't keep. Some keloids can be reduced and the appearance improved. There are no guarantees. It is important to understand that the treatment is likely to require a major time commitment. You'll have to make many trips to the doctor's office.

Dr. Downie warns patients, "You have to be willing to come to the office for treatment reguarly. Otherwise it's not worth your while."

Steroid Therapy

Carla is one of Dr. Downie's patients. She developed an earlobe keloid after a piercing. Dr. Downie asked her to commit to follow-up visits, then removed the keloid. After the removal Dr. Downie injected the area with a steroid once a week for three weeks. And she instructed Carla to wear a pressure earring at night to hold down the skin and attempt to prevent the skin cells from multiplying.

Carla was lucky. Her keloid flattened quickly. Now she has steroid injections once a month. The treatment is likely to last at least another six months.

Researchers have found that in many cases, corticosteroid injections given immediately following surgery can successfully flatten the area after keloids have been removed. Because the injections must be administered on a regular schedule, you have to be willing to follow through. One injection is not adequate. You're likely to need an injection every month until there is improvement.

To restrict keloid growth between office visits, Dr. Cook-Bolden suggests applying Mederma, an over-the-counter cream that contains an onion extract developed to help scars. Dr Cook-Bolden says, "Often between appointments for the injections, the keloids will grow. It doesn't work for everyone. But in some cases, Mederma can keep the keloids from getting bigger."

Mederma also helps to lighten the darkness created by the keloid, but it may be irritating. Before you use Mederma, patch test it on a small area in the fold of your arm or leg. It's a good idea to test for three to five days to see if there is a reaction. If your skin does react, please don't use it.

We don't want to leave the impression that surgically removing a keloid and using steroid therapy always works. It doesn't. The keloids often grow back anyway. But in many cases, this a good way to keep the growth of the keloid down so that it's neither uncomfortable nor disfiguring.

Laser Treatment

Laser surgery is another possibility for treating keloids. We describe how the laser works in chapter 29 on stretch marks and scars (see pages 262–264). But the laser used to treat keloids is often the same laser we use to treat stretch marks.

Again, we must caution you to check the credentials of the person who will perform the laser treatments. There have been too many disastrous results. And with the sensitivity of your skin, and your tendency to form keloids, you cannot afford to take any chances. In the wrong hands, the laser can easily burn and scar your skin. Make sure that your physician is a board-certified dermatologist or plastic surgeon. And be certain that the doctor understands the problems of skin of color.

In a recent study, Dr. Cook-Bolden and other researchers found that the Vbeam, or pulsed dye laser, is effective for reducing and flattening keloids. This laser specifically targets the blood supply in the keloid. Whenever a wound is healing, blood increases in the area. In the case of a keloid, there's too much healing. Remember, when keloid-prone skin heals, too many cells are produced. When you cut off the blood supply, the extra cells can't keep growing. Without the extra cells, little or no keloid forms. The laser action also causes the thick skin to contract and flatten.

The sooner you treat a keloid with a laser, the better. "It's a good idea to begin laser treatment as soon as you notice the scar and as early as two weeks after a surgical procedure," Dr. Cook-Bolden advises.

Laser treatment also requires a time commitment. It may take a treatment once a month for twenty months or more to reduce the keloid. Some people may begin to see results after three treatments, and others won't see an improvement until much later. It really depends on your skin.

COST

Treatments generally cost between $250 and $375 for each session depending on the size of the keloid, the skill of your doctor, and where you live. The cost of treating a very large keloid could be as high as $1,000. But because some people need repeated treatments, it is possible that your doctor will adjust the fees to make it more affordable.

Again, the laser scar surgery is effective for many people. But it is not a certain cure for everyone.

Radiation Therapy

If a keloid is very large and persistent, a doctor may combine radiation therapy with another treatment. Radiation therapy should not be the first choice, and it is not necessarily a good choice for everyone. With radiation, there is some risk of developing skin cancer in later years. Nonetheless, some studies show that radiation is effective when used immediately after a keloid is removed surgically.

Carolyn visited Dr. Downie looking for help for terrible keloids on her cheeks. "She had an accident. People called her elephant woman and she was very upset. I arranged for her to have surgery and radiation treatment at the Mayo Clinic in Rochester, Minnesota," Dr. Downie says.

After surgery to remove the keloids, doctors immediately irradiated the area. Carolyn also received a specially fitted pressure mask that she wore twenty-four hours a day for five months. The surgery, radiation, and pressure treatments have worked; the keloids have not grown back.

The Bottom Line

We wish we knew more. And we hope that in the not-too-distant future, scientists will unlock the mystery of the keloid. Until then, you can control the growth of most keloids, if you are willing to undergo the therapy and put in the time. It is definitely worth the effort.

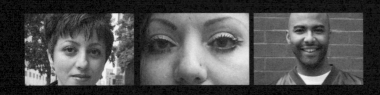

Keratoderma

CHAPTER 22

IF YOU'VE NOTICED THICKENING OF THE SKIN ON THE PALMS OF YOUR hands or the soles of your feet, you may have a medical condition called *keratoderma*. Although this is not specifically a disease related to skin of color, we see it frequently in African-Americans, Caribbean-Americans, and Latinos. It is also common among people whose families are from the Mediterranean, and it is particularly common in men.

Because many people with skin of color are often misdiagnosed, you should know how to recognize this condition. Most keratodermas are benign but can be unslightly.

Why It Happens

This is an uncomfortable problem that's usually hereditary. Look at your relatives. Someone in your family probably has the same thickening of the palms and soles of the feet. And your parents may have first noticed the thickening on your body when you were an infant. Keratoderma can appear before a person is two years old, although there are types of the disease that may develop suddenly at any time later in a person's life. We also think that keratoderma is aggravated by the constant trauma of manual labor or the use of strong chemicals.

With keratoderma, there's likely to be slight redness around thickened skin. Although keratoderma usually appears on the hands and feet, it can occur on the elbows and knees. It may also make your nails thicker than normal.

The very thick skin may make it difficult to walk, and even to hold things. Affected areas are very sensitive to cold. Your soles and palms may feel very hard in the winter months, when they can be particularly painful.

In skin of color, keratoderma may be confused with other conditions. This confusion can have dangerous consequences.

FACT: *Most people with thickened soles and palms do have keratoderma. It's a condition that requires your attention and management.*

When Anthony visited Dr. Downie's office for the first time, he showed her the thickened skin and a wartlike growth on the bottom of his right foot. Anthony told Dr. Downie that another doctor had previously diagnosed him with keratoderma. But Anthony was concerned about the persistent bleeding and the cracking skin. It wasn't healing.

A biopsy confirmed Dr. Downie's suspicion. She discovered Anthony had a slow-growing verrucous carcinoma, a variety of squamous cell cancer.

Because of the delay in the proper diagnosis, the cancer was deep in the sole of Anthony's foot. The surgery to remove it was complicated, and a significant portion of the sole of his foot had to be removed. If the first doctor had been familiar with skin of color, he might have spotted the cancer and Anthony's surgery might not have been as traumatic.

Anthony's case is somewhat unusual. Most people with thickened soles and palms do have keratoderma. It's a condition that requires your attention and management.

Remedies

What You Can Do on Your Own

The natural tendency is to pick and scratch the thick skin. Please don't do that. We see many patients who have picked their skin raw. The skin becomes infected and swollen, making the movement of hands and feet very difficult. Severe infections may require hospitalization and we don't want you to get to that point.

The alpha and beta hydroxy acids, which we describe in chapters 2 and 7, are useful for keratoderma, but you'll generally need higher-strength alpha and beta hydroxy acids to make a difference. These natural acids help to speed the natural shedding of dead skin cells. And along with retinol products containing vitamin A, they can also boost the new skin cell production. 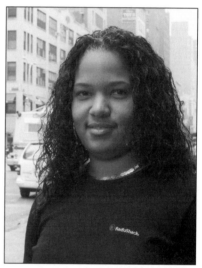 Although over-the-counter products may not be totally effective, they can provide a little extra help to the affected areas of your skin.

A wide variety of creams and lotions are sold over the counter in drugstores and beauty supply shops. Alpha Glycolic and Alpha Hydrox are readily available. But they are relatively mild, and you may need the more potent prescription-strength remedies.

Moisturizers are also essential. The softer you keep the thickened skin, the better. Moisturizers containing milk-based, lactic acids are particularly good. LactiCare, LAC-HYDRIN, and Amlactin are strong moisturizers. Jergens Ash Relief Moisturizer with beta hydroxy acid can also be helpful.

A Doctor's Guidance

A knowledgeable doctor can also help you reduce the thickening of the skin. Typically a doctor would recommend stronger alpha and beta hydroxy acids than are available over the counter. It is possible that the doctor will use the solutions in a chemical peel or prescribe creams to be applied in the morning and at night.

Typically a doctor would recommend stronger alpha and beta hydroxy acids than are available over the counter. It is possible that the doctor will use the solutions in a chemical peel or prescribe creams to be applied in the morning and at night.

A doctor might also prescribe Tazorac Gel. It is one of the most effective retinoids, vitamin A derivatives that help to renew the skin. Tazorac Gel can help shed dead skin cells and boost the production of new, healthy cells.

In very severe cases, it is possible that a doctor will prescribe an oral retinoid such as Soritane to attack the problem from the inside out. This is a strong prescription that requires monitoring by a physician. You'll need to have blood tests every month to make sure that the drug is not negatively affecting you.

Additionally, some moisturizers are only available with a prescription, including LAC-HYDRIN 12 percent and Vanamide with 40 percent urea.

The Bottom Line

Keratoderma is a medical condition with no real cure, but there are many ways to ease the thickening of the skin and accompanying discomfort.

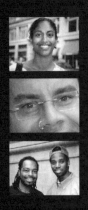

Keratosis
Pilaris

CHAPTER 23

YOU MAY CALL THOSE SMALL RAISED BUMPS ON YOUR UPPER ARMS "chicken skin." But you may also have a medical condition called *keratosis pilaris*. This ailment afflicts all skin colors and skin types, but it particularly stands out on Asian, olive, and dark skin.

And if you are like Karen, you are very self-conscious about it: "I have what so many black Americans have. There are very small dots in the hair pores on my arms and legs. The dots become raised and discolored and give my skin a rough texture. As a woman looking for a man, I can't tell you how upsetting this is. What can I do about it?"

We want to say, "We can make them all go away." Unfortunately, we can't, but we can tell you how to reduce them and make them much less obvious.

Why It Happens

We think that keratosis pilaris is related to eczema and a family history of allergies and itchy skin disorders. The latest research places the blame on genetic patterns, but the research isn't conclusive.

A lot of us must share the same gene. An estimated 40 million adult Americans suffer with keratosis pilaris. Children usually develop the first bumps before they are ten years old, although an adult may wake up one day to be unpleasantly surprised by

> FACT: *An estimated 40 million adult Americans suffer with keratosis pilaris.*

the series of small bumps on the upper arm, the front of the thighs, the back, or possibly on the cheeks.

When the bumps appear, the body is producing too much of a protein called *keratin*. The keratin clogs the pores, those small openings from which the hair comes out of our skin. The result is a tiny bump that sometimes has coiled hair twisted inside. These extra keratin proteins usually travel in packs, so instead of one bump, you get a gathering of bumps.

Cold weather brings drier skin, which in turn seems to bring out the keratosis pilaris and make it worse. You may not have any symptoms during the summer months but have a recurrence during the winter.

There are a few things you can do to help.

Remedies

What You Can Do on Your Own

Treating your skin *gently* is important here. We've seen people buy strong soaps to scrub away these bumps. And we've heard others talk about buffing the skin or using loofahs. For skin of color, that's not the

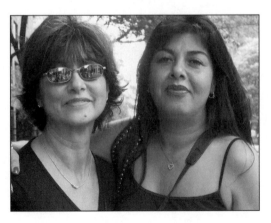

way to go. You'll still have the bumps, and you are likely to have dark marks as well as a result of the trauma to the skin.

Soap and cleansers can make a big difference. Try mild soaps like Dove or Oil of Olay. Cetaphil Cleansing Soap and Vanicream cleansers are also good. These products are less likely than other cleansers to dry out your skin. Preventing dry skin and moisturizing it are key factors in keeping keratosis pilaris under control.

Our skin loses moisture all of the time, and we have to replenish it.

The moisturizers we've mentioned will help retain moisture. But moisturizers that contain humectants will actually attract moisture to your skin. Any over-the-counter moisturizers that contain alpha and beta hydroxy acids have these humectant properties.

Alpha hydroxys and beta hydroxys also renew the skin by helping dead skin cells slough off. Washes containing hydroxy acids can be helpful, but you must use a moisturizer immediately after you use one of these washes. Some moisturizers contain natural acids and they can be beneficial. Moisturizers with milk-based lactic acid are particularly good. These include: LAC-HYDRIN, LactiCare, and AmLactin.

> FACT: *This is one instance where a little sunshine may be helpful. The sun helps to stimulate production of vitamin D, which can also diminish the keratosis pilaris. But it is important to wear a sunblock with UVA and UVB protection.*

Over-the-counter products, however, may not be strong enough to help you. Although keratosis pilaris is not a debilitating disease, you may want to a see a dermatologist who can help you create a good program for managing the problem.

In the meantime, this is one instance where a little sunshine may be helpful. The sun helps to stimulate production of vitamin D, which can also diminish the keratosis pilaris. But it is important to wear a sunblock with UVA and UVB protection.

A Doctor's Guidance

A dermatologist can design a plan with a number of complementary therapies. One procedure boosts the work of another. Initially a dermatologist is likely to recommend a series of chemical peels with the alpha and beta hydroxy acids to even your skin tone and flatten the bumps. We describe the way the peels work in chapters 2 and 7. They work they same way for keratosis pilaris.

Beta hydroxy acids are particularly effective. Dr. Cook-Bolden uses a series of beta-lift peels on her patients to smooth out the roughness, decrease the discoloration, and make the pores less obvious. "I like beta hydroxy acid because it has anti-inflammatory properties that decrease the appearance of the bumps," Dr. Cook-Bolden says.

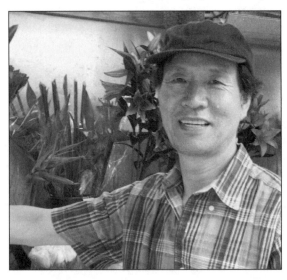

The peels are especially useful when they are combined with microdermabrasion, which helps to remove dead skin cells. We fully describe how microdermabrasion works in chapter 2, "Acne."

In addition, a doctor may prescribe a retinoid like Retin-A Micro Gel, which speeds up the process of shedding dead skin cells. Equally important, retinoids boost the production of collagen, which gives the skin a nice texture. Along with the retinoid, the doctor might prescribe a potent alpha hydroxy cream and a strong moisturizer.

The Bottom Line

Aggressive, rough action aimed at getting rid of keratosis pilaris can aggravate the condition and create other problems. That's why it is a good idea to make peace with your skin and create a systematic plan to deal with the bumps in order to minimize the flare-ups.

Laser, Light, and Radio Frequency Skin Rejuvenation

CHAPTER 24

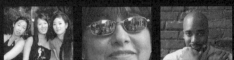

THIS IS A TRICKY SUBJECT. EVOLVING TECHNOLOGY HAS CREATED new ways to treat medical conditions and make our skin look better. These techniques are valuable for people with skin of color. In the hands of a skilled, certified doctor, lasers, light sources, and radio frequency devices are important tools for skin repair and renewal. In the hands of an untrained or unlicensed person, they can be dangerous weapons.

Doctors call these procedures *nonablative techniques.* It's a complicated way of saying that the procedures have an effect underneath the surface of the skin without cutting, burning, or deliberately damaging the outer layer of the skin. The procedures rejuvenate the skin by stimulating and remodeling collagen below the surface and stimulating the growth of new skin cells. Lasers and light sources are used to decrease superficial scarring, to smooth the skin, to improve acne breakouts, fade fine lines, and sometimes to dissolve tiny red capillaries and fade dark marks. The newest developments involve the use of radio frequency waves to stimulate collagen and tighten sagging skin.

Many people want to improve their appearance but are wary of the technology. Patrick, for example, asked us a sensible question in an e-mail: "Is laser technology advanced enough at this point to treat dark skin with minimal effects after the procedure?"

The answer is yes. The appropriate laser in the hands of a trained doctor can be safe for skin of color. There are also many nonphysicians offering laser services. We strongly advise against using anyone except a qualified physician.

Laser Skin Rejuvenation

How It Works

Laser stands for *l*ight *a*mplification by *s*timulated *e*mission of *r*adiation. The laser creates energy in the form of a coherent beam of light. The energy created by the light can be harnessed in many ways by varying the length and the intensity of the beam. It is used widely in science, medicine, and technology.

Specific lasers use specific colors of light to cut or remove the skin, close the blood vessels, or eliminate hair follicles. And other lasers can be used to stimulate the collagen that gives the skin its texture without harming the surface of the skin.

When any laser beam interacts with skin tissue, the water in the cells absorbs the heat. The heat can do damage, or it can stimulate the skin cells to make their own repairs. This is where the nonablative lasers come in. They use a long wavelength of light that passes through the epidermis, the outer layer of the skin, without harming it. The energy is directed to the inner layers of skin. This is particularly important for skin of color. The laser light targets color and is absorbed by color as well as by water, and this is why lasers that use a longer wavelength are generally safer for dark skin.

With earlier carbon dioxide (CO_2) lasers, great damage was done to skin of color because the dark melanin, or pigment, in the skin attracted and absorbed the laser light and heat. The results were often severe burns, discoloration, and permanent loss of pigment, often resulting in stark white patches and scarring.

Jessica e-mailed us about that very problem: "I had laser surgery with a CO_2 laser and it burned my skin. Now I have white patches where the doctor used the laser."

In light skin that doesn't normally have very active pigment cells, using a CO_2 laser to peel the outer two to three layers of skin is usually beneficial. Light skin is more likely to renew itself without forming blotches or scars, though the skin may be pink for several months to years after the procedure.

Skin of color reacts differently. The very active pigment cells work overtime when the skin is damaged or even mildly irritated. In most cases, the CO_2 laser is too intense for dark skin, because it interacts negatively with the pigment cells.

Dr. Cook-Bolden warns, "The CO_2 laser is not the best laser for rejuvenating skin of color. I've seen many patients with permanent scars because the CO_2 laser was used on them. I steer clear of it."

According to the American Society for Dermatologic Surgery, the wrong kind of laser procedures are often performed. That's why it's a good idea to do your homework before you sign up for any laser treatment.

A Doctor's Guidance

The Right Kind of Laser

"The right kind of laser in the right hands can help to renew your skin. A nonablative laser has a long enough beam to work below the surface without damaging the melanin," Dr. Downie says.

Laser energy is directed through the epidermis, the outer layer of skin, into the dermis, the inner layer of skin. Energy, or heat, from the laser stimulates the natural collagen, which gives the skin its texture and fullness. The activated collagen responds by renewing itself and gradually plumps up the skin to fill out shallow or superficial scars and fine lines. Laser energy also stimulates the production of new skin cells, minimizing surface blemishes and thickening the skin in a good way.

We like to use the nonablative procedure for fine lines and shallow scars, although it doesn't work as well on very deep lines and furrows. If you've suffered from severe acne, the laser treatments can make the rough, shallow pits in the skin smoother by stimulating the collagen. The laser also helps with acne treatments. It works by slowing down the oil produced by the sebaceous glands. It also helps to eliminate the tiny red capillaries.

"We've also found that if you are not overweight," Dr. Downie says, "the nonablative technique can rejuvenate an aging neck without surgery. The stimulated collagen helps plump up skin and reduce the stringy bands and lines on your neck while firming the skin."

> FACT: After the laser treatment, the cells feel the effects of the stimulation for more than four weeks. During this time, the collagen is building up and subtly filling out the top layers of the skin.

The results are not immediate. After the laser treatment, the cells feel the effects of the stimulation for more than four weeks. During this time, the collagen is building up and subtly filling out the top layers of the skin. Typically a doctor will give you one treatment every two to four weeks. And it may take six or more treatments before you see a difference. The level of improvement varies from person to person.

Remember that the newly stimulated collagen will diminish only with wear and tear. That means you have to treat your skin *gently* and protect it from the sun. It is also a good idea to begin a regimen of topical creams including alpha hydroxy acids, retinoids, and other products your doctor might recommend.

Doctors are combining therapies with nonablative laser treatment. A doctor might combine laser treatments with microdermabrasion. Dr. Cook-Bolden says, "I often perform microdermabrasion before a laser rejuvenation procedure to prime the collagen and get the process moving." We describe the benefits of microdermabrasion in chapter 2. In some cases, a doctor may use the laser to stimulate collagen in the neck and also inject the area with Botox, which we describe in chapter 4.

The Doctor's Procedure

A certified, trained doctor will inquire if you have a history of keloids, herpes, warts, or diabetes, or an autoimmune system disorder. The doctor may decide that it's not safe for you to have a laser procedure. If you have herpes, the doctor will prescribe antiviral medications before the surgery to make sure that you do not have an outbreak.

You'll have to discontinue prescription medications like Vaniqa for hair reduction, or a retinoid for acne treatment for a short time. And if you've been using alpha or beta hydroxy products, you may be instructed to take a short break from using the products. Your doctor may also advise you not to use aspirin or other blood thinners during the week prior to treatment.

It is best to test the laser on skin of color before a full-blown treatment. It is important to see how your skin will react to specific wavelengths. "You can have thirty people with the same skin color,"

IMPORTANT: *"You can have thirty people with the same skin color,"* Dr. *Cook-Bolden says, "and each one will respond differently to the laser. I always test first."*

Dr. Cook-Bolden says, "and each one will respond differently to the laser. I always test first."

Before the actual treatment a cooling gel may be applied, and you'll be asked to wear eye protection. The doctor will apply the tip of the handheld laser instrument to individual sections of your skin. You may feel a short, rubber-band-like snap as the laser's energy is directed at the area. The doctor modulates the energy according to what your skin can tolerate. The treatment is surprisingly quick and may last five to fifteen minutes.

COST

Treatment prices vary depending on the skill of the doctor, where you live, and the type of laser that's used. Prices for each laser session may range from $300 to $1,500. Some doctors will work out a plan to reduce the cost if you have multiple sessions.

Light Treatments

LEDs—Light Emitting Diodes

A variety of new nonlaser light treatments exist that are improving skin tone and texture. The newest system is based on technology NASA pioneered to grow plants in space. Oddly enough, it is something many of us see every day. The LEDs—or Light Emitting Diodes—that light up your dashboard and your alarm clock are being used to stimulate collagen and skin cells. Researchers say in order for LEDs to have a cosmetic benefit they must be calibrated to a specific frequency. Several manufacturers are developing LED devices that can penetrate the skin without harming the surface.

Gentle Waves is an LED device developed by Dr. David McDaniel, who coined the term *photomodulation* to describe the way it works. Using less than 25 watts of light, the diodes stimulate skin cell regeneration and produce collagen and elastin proteins that smooth and plump up the skin. Researchers and doctors are enthusiastic about the treatment because they believe LEDs can penetrate the skin deeply and treat broader areas than the laser.

At a treatment session you'll wear a pair of goggles to protect your eyes as you sit in front of a small panel of blinking lights emitting thousands of diodes. You are unlikely to feel anything during the thirty-five-second treatment; you may feel a tingling sensation a few minutes later. After eight of these twice-weekly sessions, researchers report that there is an improvement in skin tone and a reduction in fine lines.

This treatment is not yet approved by the FDA, and some doctors are unconvinced about its effectiveness. LED treatment is unlikely to help people with deep wrinkles and lines, who are instead candidates for face-lifts.

COST
A series of treatments is likely to cost $1,000 to $1,500.

Intense Pulsed Light
Intense pulsed light treatments are also used for rejuvenation. IPL technology is a nonlaser treatment that uses light to penetrate the surface of the skin and stimulate collagen and skin cells. When collagen is stimulated, the surface skin looks smoother and healthier. The treatment may also reduce dark marks and clear acne spots.

The treatments are performed in a doctor's office. The doctor uses a wandlike instrument to administer bursts of light that are generated and controlled by a computer system. You may feel as if you are being zapped by a rubber band as the light works on the skin. Treatments last from five to fifteen minutes, and you may have some redness or swelling, which should disappear in a few hours.

Improvement in the skin occurs gradually over a four- to six-week period as the collagen and skin cells renew. You may need four to five treatments to achieve the results you want.

COST

A single IPL treatment may cost $400. Frequently doctors will arrange a package price for a series of treatments.

Radio Frequency Waves

Radio frequency wave treatment is one of the newest developments in skin care. Doctors are using radio frequency waves to stimulate the body's natural collagen and tighten the skin without cutting or wounding the surface. Although these are the same kind of radio waves that bring us music and talk, they are uti-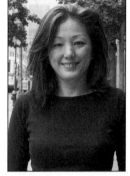lized on a much lower frequency for skin rejuvenation. The FDA has approved the use of a radio frequency wave device called Thermage for treating wrinkles around the eyes. But a number of doctors are also using the device to tighten skin on the lower face and neck.

Researchers discovered that when heat is applied to the fibrous bundles of collagen that give our skin shape and texture, the collagen responds by contracting and ultimately tightening the surface skin. Mitchell E. Levinson, vice president of research and development at Thermage, says, "The technology works in two stages: First, the heat generated by the radio frequency waves causes the bundles of collagen under the surface of the skin to unravel and shrink. As these bundles of collagen become shorter, the skin tightens." The second phase begins as the body responds, to what essentially was a wound, and the collagen heals. Levinson says, "The damaged collagen is renewed and even more collagen is produced. The skin tightens and the overall look is improved."

This treatment is new, and doctors are studying the best way to use it. Dr. Roy Geronemus, a recent president of the American Society for Dermatologic Surgery, is enthusiastic about the procedure. He says, "For the first time we have something that can tighten the skin without cutting. There are indications that using radio frequency technology we can perform a nonsurgical face-lift."

The Doctor's Procedure

The procedure is performed in the doctor's office. The treatment is painful. Before the treatment a topical anesthetic such as EMLA is applied to the area. You'll also be given a mild sedative. The doctor uses a handheld instrument that delivers the radio waves to the target area. The tip of the instrument contains temperature sensors and alternately applies a cooling agent so that the skin doesn't burn. But as the doctor moves the instrument from place to place on your skin, the nerves respond to the heat and you feel it. The treatment generally lasts about thirty minutes. You are likely to be red and swollen after the procedure. There are also likely to be bumps under the skin. Immediately after the treatment, you'll be given ice to help reduce the swelling. The redness should subside within two to twenty-four hours. Most of the bumps will disappear within a few hours. Your jaw or the area treated may feel tender for a week after the procedure. Most of the swelling should subside within a week. But it is possible that some bumps, actual areas of swollen fat, may remain for a longer period of time. Even with the slight swelling and discomfort, you should be able to return to normal activities immediately.

The effectiveness of the treatment varies from person to person.

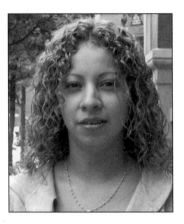

Not everyone who has had the treatment has seen an improvement. Some people see results right after the treatment. But for most it is a gradual process. It may take three to six weeks, but more likely as long as six months before the collagen contraction and replacement is complete. It's not clear how long the results last, but doctors believe you may benefit from the procedure for at least one year. Usually only one treatment is required. Some doctors are experimenting with a second treatment to see if there are additional benefits.

We do want to warn you that if you have extremely saggy skin, radio frequency wave treatment will not replace a face-lift. In addition, because the technology is new and evolving, doctors are still studying the long-term effects.

Researchers are also exploring the possibility that this may be an effective treatment to fight some acne breakouts.

COST

The treatment price is likely to range from $1,000 to $2,500 per session depending on the doctor and the area where you live.

The Bottom Line

If done correctly, nonablative procedures can help to restore and improve your skin. But these techniques require professional expertise, and we recommend that you check with the professional organizations in your state that certify dermatologists and plastic and reconstructive surgeons to get the names of qualified physicians. You may also contact the American Academy of Dermatology through its website at www.aad.org and the American Society for Dermatologic Surgery at www.aboutskinsurgery.com. Both organizations will provide information about qualified doctors in your area.

Liposuction

CHAPTER 25

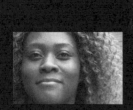

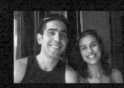

MOST OF US KNOW AT LEAST ONE SIMPLE TRUTH ABOUT OUR BODIES: fat isn't distributed evenly. We all have a layer of fat below the layers of our skin. The fat cells are the padding and protection that nature provides to arm our bodies against the outside world and to protect us from the cold. The fat also plays a role in the way we metabolize food.

But as we gain weight and add to the natural fat layer, many of us put too many fat cells in all the wrong places. A recent U.S. Surgeon General's report on obesity in America found that too many of us are overweight. According to the report, 65 percent of those in the African-American, Caribbean-American, and Latino communities simply weigh too much. In these groups, the problem is particularly acute among women.

Is it any wonder then that liposuction is one of the two most popular cosmetic procedures in the United States? Liposuction can be an issue for people with skin of color because, as with laser surgery, it can severely damage your skin if the procedure is not performed properly.

Anna is like many who've written to ask us about the safety of the procedure: "I'm a Latina with a medium complexion. I work out. But I've had two kids. I'm still young and I'd love to get rid of the fat on my hips and thighs. Is liposuction safe for someone who has color in their skin?"

It can be safe if it is performed properly by a qualified doctor with appropriate training. There are many horror stories about people who have had botched liposuction procedures by unqualified doctors—and by people who are not doctors at all. Beware of so-called clinics and spas where unlicensed, untrained individuals perform liposuction at cut-rate prices. You may be tempted by the offer of a bargain. But it is not worth the risk.

Having said that, we think that liposuction can be very effective for some people. But anyone with skin of color must be very careful because the surgery can damage the appearance of the skin and cause internal damage.

How It Works

Put a man and a woman side by side; the man's not likely to have fat thighs or a fat backside. Women's fat cells tend to migrate toward their thighs and backsides. Men's fat cells are usually a little bit more evenly distributed. If they collect in one place, it's likely to be smack in the middle of the stomach.

The way your fat cells are distributed is based on your genes, age, and maybe ethnicity. Once we reach adulthood, the number of fat cells we have remains the same. But as we gain weight, the cells get bigger. And as we lose weight, they shrink.

If you are very overweight, you may not be a candidate for liposuction. Doctors prefer to perform the surgery on people within 20 to 30 percent of their ideal body weight, and who have good skin elasticity. The stretched skin has to be able to spring back to the way it might have been if the fat cells hadn't been pushing it out.

The liposuction procedure itself is simply a matter of vacuuming out the fat cells in the areas where they collect and make bulges.

Because the fat cells are removed, it's unlikely that you'll get very fat in those areas again. But if you gain weight, the fat cells in other parts of your body may collect the fat that might have gone to, let's say, your thighs or buttocks. The cells can collect in such unlikely places as your upper back.

Health Factors

If you are very overweight, this procedure is not for you. A balanced weight-loss program of diet and exercise is the best way to reduce overall fat. If, after you have followed a program for an extended period of time, resistant pockets of fat remain, a doctor may consider liposuction.

Liposuction poses potential risks for some people. It can cause keloids, or thick external scars, because the skin must be punctured. There's also the possibility of internal scarring. People with a history of vascular problems or heart disease may be prone to blood clots that can form during the procedure, and diabetics generally have difficulty healing and are at risk during any surgical procedure. It is important for patients with a history of any of these conditions to obtain medical clearance. Once cleared, those patients should have the procedure in a hospital surgical suite or operating room where they can be monitored closely. For those patients without a medical condition, liposuction is often performed by doctors in sterile conditions in their office surgical suites.

A Doctor's Guidance

The Doctor's Procedure

Although a liposuction procedure looks deceptively simple, the correct technique requires the skill of a board-certified dermatologist or plastic surgeon. Usually, the doctor will have you stand up without your clothes on to mark the areas on your body where the fat will be removed. Many people find this very embarrassing. The procedure requires this step, and you must prepare yourself for this reality.

After the areas are marked, you'll lie down on the operating table with your face screened from the rest of your body. Most doctors perform this procedure using a long-acting local anesthetic. And it's likely that you'll be given either intravenous sedation or a pill to help you relax.

The doctor makes small incisions in strategic areas and injects a solution containing saline, epinephrine, and a local anesthetic. Then the suctioning begins. The doctor uses a long wandlike instrument and moves it back and forth through the fat in a circular pattern as the fat is vacuumed out. The doctor may also use ultrasound waves to loosen the fat and make it easier and quicker to remove.

Ideally, the fat is removed evenly so the end result is not bumpy or lumpy. It is difficult to tell from the outside how much fat is moving around on the inside. Even the most skilled doctor may take out too little, or too much, in an area. If that happens, don't be surprised if the doctor suggests another procedure to smooth the surface appearance.

The wounds are usually closed with absorbable sutures and covered with gauze patches to protect the areas and catch any oozing. You'll be able to move around immediately, but you may be uncomfortable. To try to prevent lumps from forming, many doctors bind the skin with wide-cloth tape. In all cases, you will have to wear a girdle-like garment continuously over the treated parts of your body for six to eight weeks. It is necessary to hold the skin down tightly so that it doesn't swell. Some swelling and bruising is normal.

And that's why it is particularly important for people with skin of color to choose the right doctor. The small incisions that are made in your skin can easily cause discoloration and ugly scars. With the ultrasound procedure there may be a higher risk of infection, internal scarring, and keloids. Potential complications in all liposuction procedures include blood clots, significant and painful swelling, infection, and permanent nerve damage.

Dr. Downie says, "It is possible that nerve damage can occur. I've had patients come to me after liposuction complaining that their buttocks were numb. In most cases, the nerves regenerate but a few patients have had permanent damage."

More typically, people with skin of color are upset by scarring after liposuction.

Donna had liposuction and at first was happy because she looked slimmer and her bulges disappeared. She became distressed when she realized that she developed keloids where the liposuction wand had entered her body. She visited Dr. Cook-Bolden for help. "This can happen, and if it does you need to treat the keloids as soon after the liposuction as possible," Dr. Cook-Bolden says. We describe the treatment for keloids in chapter 21.

COST

The costs of liposuction procedures vary widely depending on the skill of the doctor, the area where you live, and the areas of the body that are being treated. Procedures may range from $1,500 for a small section, like the upper arms, to $10,000 or more for a combination of face and body treatments.

The Bottom Line

Liposuction is one way to improve your appearance, but you must choose a doctor who will respect your skin and treat it *gently*. If you are prone to form keloids, you may form these scars even if the doctor does everything correctly.

Also be aware that liposuction won't remove cellulite. You can have a perfect liposuction procedure and still be left with cellulite. We explain why in chapter 6 on cellulite.

It is unhealthy to use a medical procedure as a substitute for a balanced diet, exercise, and a healthy lifestyle. Too many people have liposuction, then gain weight and have liposuction again and again. This is dangerous because repeated procedures put too much stress on your heart.

Beware also of the person offering to perform liposuction very cheaply; he or she may be unqualified to do it. That great deal can quickly turn into a costly, and possibly life-threatening, situation.

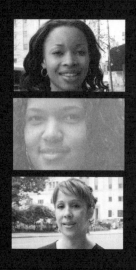

Melasma

CHAPTER 26

NOT ALL DARK MARKS ARE CREATED EQUAL. SOME ARE MORE SEVERE than others. In chapter 12, we describe the causes and treatment of dark marks. Melasma belongs in a different category. It is one of the most significant cosmetic problems that can mar skin of color.

Melasma appears as irregular brown patches on both sides of the face. They are more prominent than isolated dark marks, and they are very difficult to cover up. You may have heard about "the mask of pregnancy." That's melasma. But women who are not pregnant also develop melasma, and so do some men.

Many people recognize the problem but don't know what to do about it. Ling e-mailed us after she'd tried to erase the marks: "I'm of Asian origin and have melasma patches on my face. I tried a carbon dioxide laser. But it didn't work. Actually my skin got darker. And every time I go out in the sun, the marks darken even more."

Ling's experience, unfortunately, is typical. Melasma marks are very difficult to fade. The use of the CO_2 laser on Asian skin, and any skin of color, is risky. The CO_2 laser is one of the lasers that you should avoid, unless you are having a surgical procedure to remove a growth. The CO_2 laser is often used for cosmetic resurfacing on very fair skin, but the energy of this laser typically interacts negatively with dark skin cells.

The CO_2 laser heats the skin and burns off layers of skin cells. As it does that, the laser heat is absorbed by the melanocytes—the cells that produce pigment. The melanocytes become overactive and produce more color. That's why the melasma spots on Ling's face darkened.

There are ways to fade the melasma marks without damaging the skin. But we don't have concrete solutions for everyone because there is a lot about melasma we still don't know.

Why It Happens

We do know that melasma is genetic. If you have melasma, it is likely that another woman in your family has the same pattern of dark marks on the upper lip, the chin, or the cheeks. Although men develop it, too, it is far more common in women. And we don't know why, but Asians, Latinos, African-Americans, and Caribbean-Americans—with skin tones ranging from olive to brown—are much more likely to develop melasma than others. It is also thought that people who live in sunny climates are particularly at risk. We see melasma develop in many Latinos and Asians who either still live in southern latitudes or who grew up under the hot sun. It has historically been a problem for those who live near the Mediterranean and in the Middle East. The ancient Greeks coined a term for "the mask of pregnancy." They called it *cholasma*.

It may appear during pregnancy or during the use of oral contraceptives or hormone replacement therapy. Hormones play a key role in melasma. Researchers have isolated a molecule in the skin's melanin that resembles molecules in other hormones, and this may lead them to determine why melasma affects some women and not others. Exposure to the sun's rays during a time of hormonal fluctuation may trigger melasama.

We know how heartbreaking it can be to wake up and find these marks on your face. Embarrassment and shame are the words people use to describe the way they feel about their own appearance. They cope with the stares of strangers, and often the insensitivity of friends and relatives.

The good news is that there are things you can do to alleviate or significantly reduce melasma.

Remedies

What You Can Do on Your Own

If you have melasma, it is important to avoid the sun. The sun works a little bit like the CO_2 laser. It heats up the melanocytes and gets them rapidly producing more pigment. The deeper into the layers of skin the melasma goes, the harder it is to treat. The sun has such an impact on melasma that even if the dark marks have been completely cleared, minimal sun exposure can bring them back.

We know that it is impossible to hide in the dark, and we are not asking you to do that. But every day before you leave your house, please apply sunblock. Your skin needs an oil-free sunscreen with UVA and UVB protection, Parsol 1789, zinc oxide or titanium dioxide, and a sun protection factor of 20 to 30. Carry a tube with you so you can put it on every two hours if you are going to be outside for a prolonged period of time. And whenever you are outside, try to wear a hat to protect yourself from the sun's rays.

For a serious approach to treating melasma, you are going to need the help of a doctor who is familiar with treating skin of color.

A Doctor's Guidance

In treating melasma we have three goals: protect the skin from the sun, block the pigment production, and remove the darkened pigment. So wearing a sunblock is the first step.

We are encouraged by a combination therapy that seems to be working. Tri-Luma Cream is a prescription medication created specifically to treat melasma. The formulation is a combination of ingredients that complement each other. It contains hydroquinone, which blocks the color-producing enzyme in the melanocytes, and a retinoid, a derivative of vitamin A, that helps to shed dead, dark skin cells. The retinoid helps the hydroquinone work. And it also interacts positively with a steroid included in the formula. While the steroid works to lighten the skin and decreases the chance of irritation, the retinoid decreases the possibility that the steroid will thin the skin.

Depending on the condition of the skin and how the Tri-Luma Cream works, the doctor may also administer a series of gentle chemical peels every two to four weeks, to even out the skin tone. This treatment might also include a series of microdermabrasion sessions, and the course of treatment could last several months or several years.

Claripel is another prescription medicine that is used to treat melasma. It is a hydroquinone compound containing tyrostat, which helps to block the enzyme that makes skin darker. Claripel also contains coenzyme Q10, an antioxidant that fights the free radicals that cause fine lines and wrinkles. An added benefit is that it has full UVA and UVB protection.

EpiQuin Micro is a relatively new product containing hydroquinone and a retinol in a formula that slowly releases the ingredients into the skin to decrease the possibility of irritation. A doctor might prescribe it to treat melasma.

If the melasma is in the dermis, the layer below your epidermis, it is very difficult to treat. But the combination of treatments may make a difference. We've seen it work. Prescription fade creams, however, may irritate the skin. We recommend patch-testing a small amount twice a day in the fold of your arm. If after five days there's no irritation, it's safe to use the cream on your face.

Some health plans cover some of the cost of medication to treat melasma. Individual medications range from about $50 to more than $100.

The Bottom Line

The sun is not a friend to melasma. If you use the medication and still go out without a hat and sunblock, the melasma won't get better. Put the sun at the top of your list of things to avoid.

Don't give up. We are still trying to find concrete answers to explain why melasma occurs and the best way to treat it. We are seeing some success with the new medication, microdermabrasion, and chemical peels.

It is worth a try to combine the medication, the cosmetic procedures, and sun protection; as always, we urge you to carefully coordinate with your doctor to develop the right program for you.

Moles

CHAPTER 27

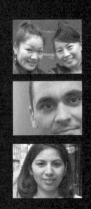

YOU MAY HAVE NOTICED A FEW TINY BLACK OR BROWN MOLES UNDER your eyes, or you may have seen them on someone else. Clusters of very small, often raised, very dark or tan moles with regular borders are common in skin of color. They are considered a medical condition called *dermatosis papulosa nigra*. Doctors see these moles on people with dark skin so frequently that they use the shorthand term DPN to describe the problem.

These dark brown moles are distinguished from other moles because they usually appear in groups under the eyes or on the cheeks, chest, and neck. They are not cancerous and not a threat to your health. But when you first spot a mole, it's important to have it diagnosed by a dermatologist to make sure that it is not cancerous.

Even if your moles are diagnosed as DPNs, a purely cosmetic problem, these clusters of moles are upsetting because they can detract from your appearance and make you uncomfortable. Often people don't know what to do and like Yoko, e-mail for help: "I'm a thirty-five-year-old Asian woman. During the last few years these tiny dark black moles began appearing on my face. I hate them. Is there any cream that I can use?"

There isn't a cream, but there are other remedies. And for some people, it is a

> **FACT:** *When you first spot a mole, it's important to have it diagnosed by a dermatologist to make sure that it is not cancerous.*

good idea to treat the moles. Nita told us she seems to see a new cluster every day: "I'm in my late twenties and about eleven years ago, these black moles started coming out on my face, chest, my neck and my back. I've never seen anyone with as many as I have. They itch. They get caught in my clothes. Sometimes they bleed. Where do they come from? Can I ever get rid of them?"

Whether you have a sprinkling of moles like Yoko or a great number of them like Nita, they can be treated.

Why It Happens

Like other problems, this one is genetic. Someone in your family probably has the same scattering of tiny black moles that you do. If you have a predisposition to develop these moles, we think that sun exposure may cause them to grow and aggravate the condition.

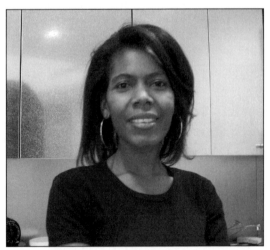

Researchers are stumped about the precise reason why your body produces these moles. Some believe that moles begin to develop in the deepest layer of your epidermis, which is called the basal layer. Scientists think that something in the genetic pattern causes a malformation of the melanocytes, the cells that give your skin pigment. These melanocyte cells form little nests that travel up to the surface of your skin as moles.

You're likely to first spot them in your teens. They'll appear under your eyes or on your cheeks, chest, or back. Don't be surprised if they multiply as you get older. Aging, however well we do it, brings out the moles. And, as with other conditions involving skin of color, the sun may make them worse.

Remedies

What You Can Do on Your Own

Creams and over-the-counter products won't eliminate the moles. You can't scrub them off. Using harsh soaps or chemicals on your face will not work. The moles will not come off. You'll only irritate the skin, activate the healthy melanocytes, and create dark marks.

Sun protection is a key factor. When outside, wearing a hat to protect your face and covering your chest and back is important. Sun protection may help limit the production of more moles. Have we talked about this before? We like sunblock-sunscreen with UVA and UVB protection, Parsol 1789, zinc oxide or titanium dioxide, and a sun protection factor of 20 to 30. It is important for you to wear sun protection whenever you are outside or driving in a car.

It's not a good idea to try to remove the moles yourself. People attempt to pull or pick them off. "Discoloration is a very big risk when you start pulling at these moles by yourself," Dr. Cook-Bolden says. "Often people try to remove them, and they get infections followed by severe discoloration."

A knowledgeable doctor can help you.

A Doctor's Guidance

A dermatologist who understands skin of color will take this condition seriously. It is likely that if you don't have a history of keloids, the doctor will easily remove them in the office. Even if you do produce keloids, a doctor may remove one or two small moles near the hairline as a test. If you heal without scarring, the doctor can move on to another series of moles. Only ten to twenty moles are removed in a single session, so your commitment to follow through and keep appointments with the doctor is really important.

If your moles appear in clusters on your cheeks, the doctor will remove a few on one side and a few on the other during several visits. It is likely that the doctor will do this with an electric needle, scalpel, or special dermatological scissors.

Removing the moles may sting a little bit, as Dr. Downie well knows. Although she's performed this procedure thousands of times

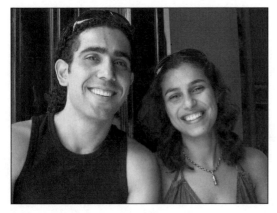

for others, in removing a few moles from her own face, she was surprised by the stinging.

After the moles are removed, the doctor is likely to administer a series of light chemical peels. We describe this process in chapter 7 on chemical peels and chapter 2 on acne. The chemical peels will help to even your skin tone and speed the formation of healthy new skin cells.

The Bottom Line

You don't have to suffer with moles. Although a doctor can remove them, keeping them from reappearing is partly up to you. Shielding your face and body from the sun is important and can help to make a huge difference in the way you look. We think that all moles should be checked by a dermatologist. It is also a good idea to be aware of cancer warning signs: if a mole changes shape, develops irregular edges, turns several colors, becomes very tender, or starts to bleed, you should see a dermatologist immediately. It may turn out to be a harmless mole. But you don't want to take any chances.

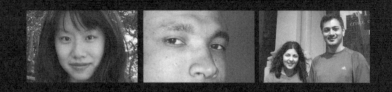

Nails

CHAPTER 28

CONSIDERING THE NUMBER OF NAIL SALONS IN OUR NEIGHBORHOODS, malls, and even out-of-the-way places, a visitor from another planet might think we're nail crazy. And in a way we are; fingernails are a fashion accessory for many of us. Whether they are simply manicured, covered with acrylics, or extended with tips and covered with flashy designs, your nails say a lot about you.

When you extend your hand for handshake, put your hands on the table, or pick up a glass to drink, your nails stand out. Our toenails, exposed by sandals or open-toed shoes, also tell a little story.

For centuries people buffed their nails and used natural dyes to stain them. Nail color told their stories, too. The rich wore polish. Ming Dynasty royals in China in 3000 B.C. painted their nails black and red. Cleopatra colored her nails a deep red, and Egyptian and Roman warriors colored their nails before their big battles. It wasn't until the twentieth century that nail polish became trendy in a big way. Cosmetic manufacturers borrowed the technology used to create car paint and invented nail polish. Red nail polish first appeared in 1925, and in 1932 the founders of Revlon introduced a nonstreaking nail polish. Since then refinements and new developments have made a vast array of products available.

As with every good thing, there's a downside. Improper nail care can lead to infections and unsightly conditions. Often we use polish, acrylics, and tips to hide problems. But it's possible that your nail care is actually creating a problem.

Kim wrote to us about a very familiar concern: "I think I've ruined my nails. I get a manicure every week, but my nails are stained yellow. Is there any hope that they'll ever be right again?"

Kim's nails may not be ruined, and returning them to their natural color is possible and may not take that long.

Santos, however, wrote to us about a more difficult problem: "Because of my work, my hands are in water all day. And my nails are a mess. They are brittle and splitting all of the time. Sometimes my cuticles get red and swollen."

What both Kim and Santos describe could happen to anyone, even if you are a regular at a nail salon. We like nail salons. We use them. But care must be taken to ensure that the nails are treated properly.

FACT: *"Often women who have regular manicures and get the most spectacular acrylics have serious bacterial or fungal infections underneath the glamorous-looking nails,"* Dr. Downie says.

"Often women who have regular manicures and get the most spectacular acrylics have serious bacterial or fungal infections underneath the glamorous-looking nails," Dr. Downie says. "This is really a big issue, and it is important to make sure that your nail salon is using proper techniques so your nails are not damaged or infected."

Why It Happens

Nails are relatively hard. But because they are made up of skin cells, they need to be treated as *gently* as the rest of your skin. The nail is a collection of specialized, protein-filled skin cells that grow out of deep folds in our fingers and toes. As the cells multiply they press together and flatten and eventually die. But the collection of cells forms a plate.

And as the plate gets bigger, it pushes forward and becomes the nail at the tip of your finger or toe.

It's a slow process. Starting from scratch, a new fingernail is formed completely in six to eight months. Toenails grow about three times more slowly. But as you may have noticed, in the summer months fingernails and toenails grow faster. Scientists haven't been able to figure out why.

In any season, your nails are healthy if they are hard, smooth, and slightly curved. Maybe you remember how they looked when you were a child. Age and the things we do to nails change their texture, color, and sometimes their shape. As we get older, our nails develop ridges and may turn slightly yellow. We also think that genetics plays a role in the formation of ridges, discoloration, and other problems that affect the nails.

Nail Care

Basic manicures and pedicures, whether performed by a salon or yourself, are necessary nail care, but they have to be done right.

Consider how you file or try to shape your nails as they are cut. Ideally, your nail should be trimmed straight across. It's best to trim when the nail is moistened and soft so it doesn't crack or split. Filing straight across, without digging into the corners, helps to maintain a healthy nail.

Although manicurists love to cut cuticles, it is not a great idea. If your cuticles are pushed back, it should be done *gently*. Abused cuticles frequently lead to ugly hangnails and difficult-to-cure fungal infections.

> **TIP:** *Ideally, your nail should be trimmed straight across. It's best to trim when the nail is moistened and soft so it doesn't crack or split.*

Jin Soon Choi of Jin Soon Natural Hand and Foot Spas in New York says, "Only nails, hangnails, and the sides of the cuticles should be trimmed. Never cut the base of the cuticle. Push back the base firmly with an orange stick or cuticle pusher, and trim the sides of the cuticle with a clean manicure scissors."

Nail polish actually helps the nails. "Polish gives added protection to the nails," says manicurist Marianne Diaconescu of New York's Pierre Mcihele salon. "It's like wearing a protective shield on each finger." Nail polish helps protect the nail from the environment and from soaps and detergents, and it seals in moisture. Your nails are likely to feel better with nail polish on them because they are less brittle and less prone to breaking or splitting.

But nail products can also be harmful. Nail polish remover dries out the nails and should be used sparingly once a week. Polishing without a base coat discolors the nails, and quick-dry polishes are very drying and can also cause discoloration. "Quick-dry polishes are a problem," Dr. Downie says. "They often cause nails to yellow."

Some nail polish colors also cause stains. As Kim learned, red polishes stain the nails and make them yellow, particularly if you wear the polish for more than seven days. The stain will fade if you don't polish your nails with a dark red color for several weeks.

Yellow nails are also caused by smoking, harsh chemicals, household detergents, fungal infections, lung problems, and aging; in some cases the stain can be reduced.

Allergies

Whether you realize it or not, you may be allergic to nail polish. It's possible that if you have itchy patches on your eyelids, the nail polish is to blame. Toluene, a central ingredient in nail polish, and formaldehyde are the irritants provoking the reaction. "You don't realize how many times a day you touch your eyes. The skin on the eyelids is thin and easily irritated. Allergy-prone people need to be careful. When you touch your eyes, if you are wearing polish or have just used remover there's a good chance you'll have a breakout on the lids," Dr. Downie says.

If you suffer from nickel allergies that cause eczema, there's another issue to consider. Many nail polish bottles have a little metal ball or metal beads inside to help stir up the polish. The metal is usually made of nickel, which can aggravate eczema.

Nail Art

Acrylics and tips are often beautiful. For some they're works of art and personal expression. But frequently, serious problems occur when they're not applied and maintained properly. Jin Soon Choi says, "We won't do acrylics. It's too easy to have problems. Infections can grow underneath the compound. You file down the real nail surface to apply the acrylic and you can hurt the real nail. There are problems when the nails grow and the acrylic loosens. In between manicures, people don't fill in the spaces between the nail and the acrylic. This open space gets irritated and infections form."

Nail tips, which are glued on the tip of the nail and covered with acrylics, present the same problem. Acrylics that are bonded under a heat lamp after they are applied also may hide an infection.

Dr. Cook-Bolden wore acrylic tips for two years. "They made my nails very weak. After I stopped wearing them, it took another two years for my nails to regain their strength," she says.

Dr. Downie isn't a fan of acrylics and tips because they conceal problems. "When women regularly cover their nails with these things, it is very common to see bacterial infections in the cuticle as well as fungal infections," Dr. Downie says.

Dr. Downie's patient Brenda regularly wore acrylics. She had persistent pain underneath her left index fingernail and she ignored it. When it started to bleed, she went to see Dr. Downie. "She didn't want to remove the acrylic, but I sent her to a nail salon to have it removed immediately. A biopsy uncovered a squamous cell skin cancer. The growth was removed and we were able to save Brenda's finger," Dr. Downie says.

Brenda's story is extreme. It's more typical to see fungal infections growing under acrylics and extensions. To make sure you don't get a fungal infection, a manicurist should apply an antibacterial, antifungal solution after cleaning, trimming, and filing. Problems also may arise when you take false nails off. If you yank at them and cause irritation, you're creating a breeding ground for a fungal infection.

Toenails

Toenails involve a separate set of issues. We beat our feet up. We stuff them into cramped shoes and squash our toes. We play sports and stress them. That's why toes and toenails change shape and may even look gnarled.

Toenails may thicken naturally as you get older. But trauma to the toenail and fungal buildup also create thickness.

Ingrown toenails often develop because of the shoes we wear, or because of the way we cut our toenails. Again, trimming each nail straight across, without digging into the corners and the skin, is the safe way to cut the nail. Sometimes it's a good idea to allow the corners to grow a little longer so toenails don't grow into the skin.

Fungal Infections

Fungal infections are very common and can affect all parts of the body.

It is also possible for fungus to form after you've used antibiotics. Antibiotics sometimes knock out the good bacteria that can fight fungus. Using steroids to reduce inflammation can also stimulate fungal growth. People with diabetes frequently develop fungal infections because the chemical imbalance associated with the disease creates a susceptibility to infection.

Fungal infections can be contagious. One person may pass a fungus to another using the same shower or walking on the same locker room floor. Similar to athlete's foot, fungal infections can develop in your fingernails and your toenails. Brittleness, thickening, peeling, and yellow or brown discoloration are signs of fungus. It may be caused by keeping your hands or your feet wet all the time.

Even if you've never had a manicurist apply acrylics or extensions, unsterilized instruments in a manicure salon can transmit fungal infection. If a salon doesn't use antibacterial and antifungal solutions and fails to clean the washing bowls and pedicure stations properly, a fungal infection can pass from one person to another. Dr. Downie says, "Make sure that bowls are washed and disinfected before you put your hands or feet in them. Many of my patients look like they have beautiful pedicures and manicures. But underneath they have terrible infections. Don't be afraid to speak up. Ask the manicurist if she's washed the bowls. This is important because the infection can so easily spread from one nail to another."

Earlier in the chapter we mentioned that Santos reported brittle nails and swollen cuticles because his job requires him to keep his hands wet.

Santos may have an infection called *paronychia*. This can be caused by a fungus or bacteria. People who work with their hands in water frequently get this infection. The signs are malformed nails and painful, red swollen cuticles. Because of the pain and the likelihood of infection, it's a good idea to see a doctor for medical treatment.

Remedies

What You Can Do on Your Own

Creating a healthy grooming routine for nails is important. If you wear nail polish and your nails are stained, removing the nail polish is the first step. Once the color is removed, it usually takes about fourteen days for the yellow to fade.

> IMPORTANT: *Creating a healthy grooming routine for nails is important. If you wear nail polish and your nails are stained, removing the nail polish is the first step. Once the color is removed, it usually takes about fourteen days for the yellow to fade.*

Be careful when using nail polish remover. Try using it only once a week. Moisturizers are beneficial for very dry nails and cuticles. You may notice that when you are at the beach or a lake, your nails seem healthier. That's because the water and the humidity in the air increase the water content of your nails without oversaturating them. Your nails are about 16 percent water. And like the rest of your body, they lose water naturally and get dry.

A good moisturizing lotion or cream can have a similar effect as the ocean air and seal moisture in the nails. We especially like moisturizers that contain humectants that attract water when you apply them to the skin or the nail. New moisturizers are being developed that have added benefits. Many now contain alpha and beta hydroxy acids and urea, which are particularly helpful. Eucerin, LAC-HYDRIN, AmLactin, LactiCare, and Carmol 20, and Jergens Ash Relief are among the products that are available over the counter. There are also more powerful prescription-strength moisturizers such as Vanamide that are particularly good for thinning thick toenails.

If your nails are very brittle, soaking your hands in water for ten to twenty minutes each night and then applying a thick coat of moisturizer before you go to bed can help. To keep the moisturizer on, wear cotton gloves or a tube sock to cover your hands. This isn't an overnight solution. It takes consistent application over several months to really see a difference.

> TIP: *If your nails are very brittle, soaking your hands in water for ten to twenty minutes each night and then applying a thick coat of moisturizer before you go to bed can help.*

Simple, commonsense practices can help you avoid fungal infections. Make sure that the manicure salon takes sanitary precautions. If you use a shower or steam bath or walk around in the locker room at your gym or health club, wear rubber sandals.

If you do contract a fungal infection or have a painful ingrown nail, it is a good idea to see a doctor.

A Doctor's Guidance

A doctor can cut an ingrown toenail and shape it properly. Any attempt to dig at it yourself may permanently destroy your nail.

Curing a fungal infection is not easy. It requires time and patience. If the infection is on your fingernails, the doctor is likely to ask you to try to keep your hands dry or use cotton gloves underneath waterproof gloves when you wash dishes or work with your hands in water. It's really important to keep the nails and hands clean. The doctor will likely recommend antifungal solutions to be used twice a day and may prescribe an oral antifungal medication.

If the fungal infection is paronychia, the doctor may prescribe oral antifungal medications as well as topical antifungal remedies and a topical anti-inflammatory solution.

Penlac Nail Lacquer is a relatively new treatment. It's a nail polish with an antifungal ingredient that must be applied every day. It takes almost a year to work. "I was skeptical about this," Dr. Cook-Bolden says. "But I do see a very good response in many patients." A doctor might also prescribe Loprox topical solution, Spectazole Cream, Mentax Cream, or Naftin Gel.

Oral antifungal medications are effective treatments, but many doctors are reluctant to prescribe them because of potentially dangerous side effects. When nothing else works, a doctor may prescribe Lamasil. It is an oral antifungal medications that decreases fungus significantly. But it can damage the liver and have other serious possible side effects. Doctors require blood tests before they prescribe this medication. Typically, you will take Lamasil for three to four months. During that time, the doctor will perform blood tests to make sure that you are not suffering from side effects and that your liver is healthy.

The Bottom Line

Enjoy your manicure and pedicure but make sure that you and the manicurist are following safe practices.

When problems arise, take care of them quickly. Most problems with fingernails and toenails can be solved. This is another example of the importance of taking the time to follow through. There are no shortcuts, particularly if oral or topical medication is necessary.

Stretch Marks and Scars

CHAPTER 29

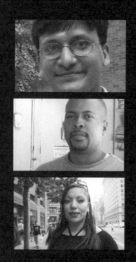

WE EXPECT SOME SCRAPES AND BRUISES IN A LIFETIME. BUT THERE ARE some marks that develop on our bodies that really stand out. If you have stretch marks or a scar, you know what we're talking about. Even if it isn't a very bad scar, doesn't interfere with your movement, and can be hidden with makeup or clothes, scars and stretch marks often make us feel self-conscious and somehow less than perfect.

Stretch marks and scars that are not keloids, or raised scars, are actually indentations in your skin. We hear regularly from people like Tina who are looking for solutions: "I started to develop stretch marks at the age of six when I began to get taller. I'm 5´4˝ and weigh 120 pounds. That's nowhere near fat. But I have stretch marks on the backs of my knees and on my upper arms running down to my elbows."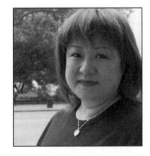

Pregnant women often find that the stretch marks creep up on them. Roxanne e-mails: "I'm a woman of color. Is there a safe and easy way to get rid of the stretch marks on my stomach that developed during my pregnancy?"

There may be ways to lighten some stretch marks and scars. New technology has improved the chances for fading them. Let's consider stretch marks first.

Why It Happens

Stretch Marks

Stretch marks appear during rapid periods of growth either upward or outward. That's probably what happened to Tina. As she grew, the skin on her limbs didn't have enough elasticity. The elastic fibers in the skin couldn't keep up with her rapid growth. In weakened areas, tiny tears occurred and the skin indented, creating stretch marks. Often stretch marks are discolored because when the pigment cells were activated by the trauma of the tiny tears, more color was produced. Over time, these areas may become lighter than the surrounding skin.

If you have a sudden weight gain or loss, you may see stretch marks. And if you are an athlete, lift weights, and are bulking up or building muscle quickly, your skin may not be able to keep pace. The result is stretch marks.

We also think that hormones play a role. As you're growing, when you're pregnant, and when you gain or lose weight, your hormones fluctuate. It's believed that estrogen levels affect the way skin cells develop and ultimately the look and texture of the skin. That may explain why women have more stretch marks than men. Women typically get stretch marks on their thighs, buttocks, stomachs, and breasts. Men tend to develop them on their backs, buttocks, and upper arms. Dr. Downie says, "We think genetics plays a big role in the development of stretch marks in both men and women."

Stretch marks are also a side effect of steroid abuse. If you are using oral steroids in an effort to enhance performance or applying powerful, topical steroid creams inappropriately to your skin, there's a strong possibility that you'll develop stretch marks.

Once you've gotten a stretch mark, it is difficult to eliminate.

Remedies

What You Can Do on Your Own

There is not much you can do on your own, and there's very little that you can do to prevent them in the first place. Dr. Downie tries to head them off in pregnant patients by suggesting that they use a moisturizer on the belly and breasts. "I tell women to apply Cetaphil moisturizer five or six times a day. The moisturizer may have some effect. But I also see people who moisturize ten times a day, and they still develop stretch marks."

When the stretch marks appear, Dr. Cook-Bolden recommends applying Mederma, an over-the-counter product that contains an onion extract, three times a day. "In some successful cases, it makes the scar or stretch mark appear smoother or less noticeable. But it's not going to work on a huge scar, and it doesn't work for everyone."

And that brings us to the problem of the traditional scar that isn't a keloid, superraised, or what doctors call *hypertrophic*. We describe the appropriate treatment for keloids in chapter 21.

Scars

A scar is the result of an injury or surgery on the skin. Severe cuts and burns damage the natural collagen that creates the skin's texture. When there's an indented scar, it means that the collagen was damaged so badly that there isn't enough to plump the skin up in that area.

Julie writes, "I'm an Asian-American woman and I have a scar on my face from an accident. Is there any cream that will help?"

Creams and lotions won't help a very deep scar. They also won't help on big surgical scars. "Women come in all the time after breast reduction surgery with very wide scars. In many cases, I've been able to reduce them with laser treatments so that they don't stand out as much. But this takes several treatments and isn't a quick process," Dr. Cook-Bolden says.

A Doctor's Guidance

The way a doctor treats your stretch marks or scars depends on your skin and how bad the problem is.

Because both scars and stretch marks are caused by a breakdown in natural collagen and elastic fibers, using a retinoid can often help create some improvement. Retinoids, like Retin-A Micro Gel or Renova, are derivatives of vitamin A. Vitamin A boosts the production of collagen. So if you catch the stretch marks or scar early enough and the scar isn't raised, it is possible that a doctor would prescribe a strong retinoid.

But it is not a sure thing. The sooner stretch marks and scars are treated, the better. Ideally, a doctor would like to see you within two weeks after the appearance of a scar.

For very superficial scars and stretch marks, a doctor might perform microdermabrasion. We describe this process, in which the top layer of dead skin is removed gently, in chapter 2 on acne. As the dead skin cells are removed, new ones take their place. Microdermabrasion also stimulates collagen production. The skin may fill out a bit, and the scarring might be lighter. It's the same principle for stretch marks.

Doctors are increasingly enthusiastic about recent advances in dermatological lasers for treating stretch marks and scars. The technology is improving constantly, making it safer to treat skin of color with a laser.

In chapter 21 on keloids and chapter 24 on laser skin rejuvenation, we explain how the laser works, and why some lasers are too dangerous to use on dark skin. Early lasers interacted negatively with the melanocytes—the pigment that gives skin color. These lasers damaged the skin and caused burns, discoloration, and scarring.

In many cases, new types of lasers can treat the skin without damaging the pigment. But Dr. Cook-Bolden warns, "You still have to be very careful. I like to go step by step. I test and test. And often I use two different lasers to see which one has the best effect."

Doctors often use a vascular laser. The laser's energy targets the blood vessels that feed the scar. The heat contracts the blood vessels. With less blood flowing to the scar, the growth is slowed. The scar is likely to shrink and fade.

Recently, using a vascular laser called the Vbeam, Dr. Cook-Bolden treated an eight-year-old who was recovering from cancer of the jaw. The surgery that removed the cancer created a huge scar on his face. It was so large and tight that it restricted his facial movement. Dr. Cook-Bolden says, "The Vbeam laser reduced and faded the scar significantly. The little boy now has normal facial movements and looks much better."

But the vascular laser is dicey for skin of color. "I've seen cases where the vascular laser actually made the scar thicker," Dr. Cook-Bolden says. That's why she also uses the Nd:Yag laser, which has a long pulse width that can be varied and directed at a specific target. The energy produced by this laser works underneath the top layers of skin to stimulate collagen production without interfering with the pigment cells.

The laser stimulation continues to have an effect on the collagen cells after the actual treatment. Collagen cells continue to react and multiply for about four weeks. That's typically when you begin to notice a change.

Your skin may respond quickly, and you may need only a few treatments. But it's also possible that you'll require twenty or more laser treatments to really improve a scar or stretch marks. And you have to be willing to follow through.

When treating stretch marks with various lasers, Dr. Downie carefully measures sections of each mark. She wants the patient to have a realistic understanding of what is being done and what is possible. Dr. Downie measures the stretch marks again two weeks after the initial treatment. "If it is an old stretch mark and after two treatments there's not a significant decrease, I'll recommend against going further. I've noticed an improvement in only about thirty percent of my patients and I don't want to create false hopes."

It's possible that along with the laser treatments, the doctor will use microdermabrasion to help even out the skin tone and stimulate collagen. With scars, a doctor may also decide to inject a steroid directly into the scar in order to flatten it.

COST

The price of laser and microdermabrasion treatments will vary depending on the skill of the doctor and the area where you live. Typically, prices for each laser treatment run between $400 and $600. Microdermabrasion generally costs between $175 and $250. But because many treatments are usually required, some doctors will reduce the fee and create a combination price. If you commit to the treatment, a doctor might charge as little as $375 for both procedures.

Light Treatment

There is a new, nonlaser treatment for scars and stretch marks that is effective for people who seek early treatment of a scar or stretch mark. ReLume Repigmentation Phototherapy is a light system that stimulates the melanocytes, restores pigment, and evens out skin tone. ReLume works on the same principle as a tanning machine, but it is safer because it does not project ultraviolet rays.

The treatment is performed in the doctor's office. Light is applied to a specific area through a handheld device attached to a small computer that generates and regulates the light. Wavelengths of energy provoke the melanocytes to produce more color and darken the lighter spots in the target areas. The treatment is quick and painless. The number of treatments depends on the severity of the problem. Typically six to twelve weekly treatments may be needed.

Areas on the face, neck, and torso seem to respond to this treatment better than other parts of the body. But again, you have a better chance of getting results if you treat the stretch mark or scar soon after it develops.

Follow-up maintenance treatments are likely to be needed.

COST

A treatment might cost $500 to $1,000 depending on the area of the body. Because multiple sessions are required, the doctor may work out a payment program that may reduce the overall cost.

The Bottom Line

It bears repeating: caution and patience are required. We are concerned about recommending medical procedures when we know that many untrained and unlicensed people are using technology incorrectly. They advertise special prices, but you may get far less than special treatment. There's the possibility of injury and disfigurement. Be careful when choosing your doctor. Make sure that you use only a board-certified dermatologist or plastic surgeon. And be sure that the doctor is familiar with treating skin of color. You can find qualified doctors on the websites of the American Society for Dermatologic Surgery, www.aboutskinsurgery.com, and the American Academy of Dermatology, www.aad.org.

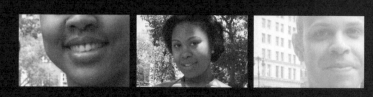

Sun
Protection

CHAPTER 30

IN EVERY CHAPTER OF *BEAUTIFUL SKIN OF COLOR*, WE MENTION THE SUN
and almost always talk about the improtance of sun protection.

We love the sun. A bright, sunny day can warm the body and
infuse the mind and spirit with a sense of great optimism. The sun
makes us happy. We love the beach. During island vacations the sun
heightens the natural beauty and contributes to the feeling that we're
visiting a special and luxurious place.

The sun is vital for all living things. Its
nourishment helps plants and animals
grow. It's also important for our good
health. The sun promotes the production
of vitamin D. We need it to absorb the calcium that's a source of bone strength. The
sun can also make you and your skin feel
better if you have medical conditions such
as eczema, psoriasis, and keratosis pilaris.

> *The sun promotes the production of vitamin D. We need it to absorb the calcium that's a source of bone strength. The sun can also make you and your skin feel better if you have medical conditions such as eczema, psoriasis, and keratosis pilaris.*

But just as the sun warms us, makes
us feel good, and is otherwise beneficial,
it is also doing a kind of devil's work.
Overexposure to the sun is probably the
biggest cause of skin damage.

No skin type is exempt. If you have the darkest pigment in your
skin and worship the sun to get even darker, you are playing a game of
Russian roulette.

We know that you don't want to, and can't always, avoid the sun. We're not suggesting that you shut yourself away, quit sports, or give up wonderful vacations. But we are saying that to have beautiful healthy skin and enjoy a healthy lifestyle, it is vital to protect the skin.

Forgive us for repeating ourselves; sun protection prevents premature aging and reduces the possibility that you'll get skin cancer. In chapter 5 on skin cancer we point out that people with dark skin *do* get the various kinds of skin cancer.

For skin of color, sun protection offers another benefit. It helps keep dark marks, moles, and other skin irregularities under control.

There's extensive misinformation about skin of color. How many times have you heard that Asian, olive, and dark skin protects you from the sun? That's true, up to a point. You do have more protection than a milky-white person from Scandinavia or the Slavic countries. But the same pigment that protects you also has the ability to react negatively to the sun. The sun can be an irritant. If your skin is already blemished, scraped, cut, or traumatized in any way, the sun can stir up the color-producing melanocytes. When these cells are stimulated, they produce more color. Your overall skin darkens, and if you've already got a mark on your skin, the sun can make it darker, too. Dark marks produced by medical conditions such as acne, moles, melasma, keloids, and scars all run the risk of growing darker. Sun protection, then, should be a part of your daily routine.

> **FACT:** *The same pigment that protects you also has the ability to react negatively to the sun. The sun can be an irritant. If your skin is already blemished, scraped, cut, or traumatized in any way, the sun can stir up the color-producing melanocytes.*

Why It Happens
How the Sun Attacks Our Skin

On some days the rays of the sun seem so visible, you think you can reach out and touch them. These golden rays piercing the blue sky with shafts of light are pretty enough to make you smile. How easily nature deceives us. These lights rays are actually beams of radiation that can play havoc with your skin.

Most often it is the *invisible* rays that can't be seen by the human eye that do the most damage. To some extent, we're protected from them. The most harmful radiation is blocked by a shield of ozone gas surrounding Earth. But this ozone layer of the atmosphere, which absorbs a portion of the ultraviolet radiation, has become thinner during the past twenty years, reducing our protection from the two primary types of ultraviolet radiation that normally pass through it.

These solar rays are called Ultraviolet-A, or UVA, and Ultraviolet-B, or UVB. These letters can make deciphering information labels on sunscreens and other products confusing and the products difficult to use.

Let us break the code.

UVA is the name for the sun's longest rays. The UVA rays tan your skin. They may not burn you right away, but they may cause redness later, particularly if you are using a tanning machine, which we don't recommend. Tanning machines deliver direct, unfiltered exposure to UVA and UVB rays and don't offer the tiniest cloud cover or bit of ozone layer to protect you.

UVA rays can, over time, make you look older. They penetrate the skin deeply and damage the DNA. UVA rays destroy the collagen and elastin cells that give your skin shape and texture. We need these protein cells to keep our skin looking fresh and springy. Your skin dries out when the collagen and elastin break down. The skin sags. Wrinkles form, and the skin looks older than it might have if the sun hadn't been working on it.

Beyond the cosmetic issues, the UVA rays can cause some skin cancers.

UVB rays are shorter and are also dangerous. UVB rays cause sunburn and are thought to be the primary cause of most skin cancers. There's no question that people with skin of color, regardless of how light or dark, can get skin cancer.

In addition, both UVA and UVB rays contribute to aging by triggering the oxygen free radical compounds that form in the body. These oxygen free radicals speed aging in your skin.

Where Sun Protection Is Needed Most

In the world's tropical climates, the sun's ultraviolet rays are always strong. These are the regions closest to the equator, the "belt" at the waistline of the earth. The tilt of the earth on its axis in relation to the sun determines how much radiation strikes areas north or south of the equator. In the Northern Hemisphere, the summer months of June, July, and August receive the brunt of the sun's rays. South of the equator, summer's bombardment from the sun occurs in December, January, and February.

The time of day, in any latitude and in any season, affects the amount of sun exposure you'll get. The sun is strongest and the radiation is most potentially damaging between ten in the morning and three in the afternoon.

Your surroundings count as well. Look at the way your skin darkens at the beach. It's not simply the sun above doing the work. The water and the sand reflect and intensify the UV radiation by 25 percent. It's as if you were sitting in the sun with two wide reflectors directed at you. The radiation is magnified.

> **FACT:** *The sun is strongest and the radiation is most potentially damaging between ten in the morning and three in the afternoon.*

Similarly, if you're skiing or snowshoeing, the reflection from the flat, white surface of snow increases the sun's radiation by 85 percent. And in the mountains, you are subject to even greater UV exposure because air is thinner at higher altitudes.

But you don't have to be at the water or on snowy mountaintop. All flat surfaces reflect the sun's rays, including concrete, tarmac, and asphalt. The parking lot at the mall reflects the sun and increases your exposure.

Is it any wonder then that we talk constantly about sun protection? We all need protection, but which product should you choose? If you're choosing a product based on fragrance, you may be making a mistake. The perfumes in those sunscreens can irritate your skin and create dark marks. Beyond the UVA and UVB issues, we also know that other jargon on the labels of these products can be baffling.

Sunscreens and Sunblocks

There are sunscreens and sunblocks. There's a difference. A sunscreen chemically absorbs UV rays. Sunblocks reflect and scatter the rays. The best products contain both sunscreen and sunblock.

In the past, many people with skin of color wouldn't wear sunblock because it left a white film on the skin and looked unattractive.

But sun protection has evolved considerably during the past ten years. New formulations have improved protection with less filminess.

A combination of UVA and UVB protection is essential.

If the label on a sun protection product says it provides UVB protection, it's likely to include water-resistant salicylates that are gentle on the skin. The other chemical for UVB protection is cinnamates, which are not water-resistant. Some people, however, are allergic to cinnamates. It is a good idea to test a small amount in the fold of your arm before applying it to your face and other parts of your body. If there is no reaction, it is safe to apply the product.

Researchers have been less successful at developing effective protection against UVA rays. But relatively recently, the U.S. Food and Drug Administration has allowed the use of Parsol 1789 in products. This chemical provides strong UVA protection.

We recommend that you look for products that also include sunblockers, such as zinc oxide or titanium dioxide. Dr. Cook-Bolden says, "Every time I tell a patient this they moan. Just recently, Tara began to develop very dark spots on her face. We went to work to fade them, but when I told her to use a sun protection cream, she said, 'I've tried them, but they make me look like a ghost.' I told her the new products are getting better."

Zinc oxide and titanium dioxide have been refined for use in sun protection products so they are not as thick or as obvious as they once were.

Many products also contain antioxidant vitamins C and E. They fight the sun-stimulated free radicals that cause aging.

Even with the best combination of all of these ingredients, the protection factor is very important. The sun protection factor, or SPF, is a standard set by the FDA to measure how long it will take you to burn while wearing sun protection. If you are wearing an SPF of 30, it will, theoretically, take you thirty times longer to burn with the product on your skin than if you are out in the sun without it.

We say this throughout *Beautiful Skin of Color*, and we'll say it again: we strongly recommend at least an SPF of 15, but we think the standard should be between SPF 20 and SPF 30 for everyone for daily use.

There is still more language on the labels that needs decoding.

A "water-resistant" product will continue to provide sun protection for forty minutes after you've been in the water.

IMPORTANT: *We strongly recommend at least an SPF 15, but we think the standard should be between SPF 20 and SPF 30 for everyone for daily use.*

But a "very water-resistant" product protects for eighty minutes. This used to be called waterproof.

Dr. Downie advises that no matter what the labels claim, "The truth is they are not really waterproof, and you lose protection when you are in the water. The rule is to reapply sun protection after you leave the water and towel dry."

Regardless of which kind of sun protection you buy, it's smart to apply it fifteen or thirty minutes before you go outside. If you're outside for a long time, reapply it every two hours. You may need to put on more lotion than you think. The best protection for the entire body requires at least one ounce of sunscreen-sunblock.

Dr. Cook-Bolden adds another caution: "Make sure that you apply it while your skin is dry and before you begin to perspire."

Creams and cosmetics that contain sunscreen are terrific. But they are not necessarily a substitute for a full-spectrum sun protection product. This kind of sun protection can be applied *before* you put your makeup on. If you are spending time outside or driving in a car, it's a good idea to use a product that combines the full range of protection. Dr. Downie says, "Many people don't realize that the sun can penetrate through a car's windshield and darken and damage the skin significantly."

Because skin of color is extremely sensitive, we recommend that you buy an oil-free sun protection product that won't clog your pores and create a climate for acne breakouts.

Sunburn

It happens. We forget to apply sun protection. We fall asleep in the sun or work in it too long without realizing that it is searing our skin. A sunburn is an inflammation of the skin that is caused by too much exposure to ultraviolet radiation. You may notice the burn immediately or even twenty to twenty-four hours later. The area of your skin is likely to be red, darker, inflamed, tender, and hot. And you can expect the skin to peel four to seven days after the burn.

Remedies

Sunburns are frequently painful, but they aren't usually life-threatening. Soothing, nonirritating creams can make you feel better. SBR Lipocream or a thin coat of Vaseline Petroleum Jelly is often effective. Taking cool baths or showers and applying a compress of Burow's solution to the sunburned area can soothe the skin. Two aspirin or ibuprofen will help to ease the pain and reduce the inflammation.

If you are very sore and the pain persists for more than a day or two, it is a good idea to see a dermatologist. The doctor is likely to prescribe stronger creams or lotions, and perhaps an anti-inflammatory to calm down the burn.

The Bottom Line

We want you to enjoy your life and also have beautiful skin. Read the labels on sun protection products to make sure that you are getting the best protection possible. We recommend an oil-free, noncomedogenic sunblock. The product should contain UVA and UVB protection, with an SPF of at least 20, as well as titanium dioxide or zinc oxide and Parsol 1789.

Tattoos

CHAPTER 31

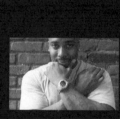
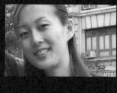
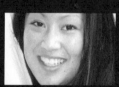

SO EASY TO GET, BUT SO HARD TO REMOVE. THAT'S THE MOST COMMON complaint we hear about tattoos. We're not foolish enough to ask, "Why did you do it?" And we won't say, "Don't do it."

We know that tattoos are a form of personal expression, and we support your right to express yourself as long as it doesn't hurt you.

People have adorned their bodies with permanent markings since the beginning of time. Today, tattoos are deeply rooted in the religious and traditional practices of many cultures.

The Bible contains accounts of tattoos in ancient Israel, along with admonitions against them, and there is evidence of tattoos on the bodies of Egyptian mummies buried in the pyramids. As we follow the tattoo trail, we see the practice spread to Africa, Asia, the South Pacific, and both Latin and North America, where Native Americans applied tattoos long before Europeans set foot on the soil.

Over the centuries, tattooing has passed in and out of mainstream culture, just like other fashion trends. This can be a problem. If the trend passes or your taste changes, you may want to remove the tattoo. Removing a tattoo is not as easy as giving away a piece of clothing that's yesterday's style.

Tattoo regret is common. We hear it from patients and in letters and e-mails like this one from Scott: "I'm really desperate. Now that I'm a businessman, the tattoos on my arms don't fit into my lifestyle. As a result of the tattoos, I don't wear short sleeves on a hot summer day. I have very dark skin. Is there any way they can be safely removed?"

Lum e-mailed with another plea we hear frequently: "I'm a twenty-four-year-old Asian female. I currently have a tattoo with my ex-boyfriend's name on my arm, and I'm dying to have it removed. The only problem is that because of my skin color, I'm afraid it will leave a scar."

Scarring and discoloration should be concerns for people with skin of color. It's an important consideration when you have the tattoo put on, and when you attempt to have it removed.

Because the pigment cells are very active in skin of color, any rough action or trauma can cause the pigment cells to create more color and leave discoloration. Also, the wrong kind of treatment can permanently remove the pigment from the skin and leave white patches.

It is possible to remove some tattoos, and fade others significantly. But they are difficult to remove entirely because the color is deeply embedded in your skin.

How It Works

A tattoo is a permanent mark of color made in the skin. Tattooing is not a superficial action that's remedied easily. Tattoo needles break through the protective barrier of the outer layers of your skin. The needles deposit color in the dermis—the deep layers of the skin. This is a serious alteration of your skin. The cells in the dermis absorb the color, and you see the result on the top layer of skin. Once the dermal cells take on the color, it's permanent.

You may not realize how deeply the color is embedded. A good artist makes tattooing look deceptively easy. Nino Desuyo at Tattoo Seen, in New York's Greenwich Village, showed us how it's done as he applied a delicate, looping tattoo of his own design to Yen's lower leg just above her ankle. It was her first tattoo.

Nino set up his workstation while Yen waited. He removed a set of five new needles that had been stored in a sterile package. He inserted them in a metal shaft that had been sterilized and then attached it to a metal tube. Nino covered the handheld, electronic tattoo machine with a plastic bag to prevent bacteria from contaminating the needles. After connecting the tube and the shaft to the machine, he looked as if he was holding a small drill.

Yen sat down opposite him. After pulling on a pair of new rubber gloves, Nino washed the lower part of Yen's leg with an antibacterial soap and shaved the area he was about to tattoo. He washed it again, dried the leg, and then pressed a stencil of his tattoo drawing on the spot. The ink transfer left the impression on Yen's skin. Nino applied A&D ointment to the skin. "It makes the needles move smoother," he said. Tattoo artists regularly use more than one needle at a time. A single needle is used only for drawing thin, fine lines.

They had both decided that a reddish-brown color would look nice on Yen's olive skin. Nino held the tattoo machine over a tiny plastic cup of reddish-brown pigment and delicately dipped the five tiny needles into the color. His foot hit the pedal, and the tattoo machine began working like a sewing machine. The color was sucked up through the tube into the needles, and in an instant, five needles moved quickly in and out of Yen's skin. Color filled the tattoo. "I don't really know how many times they go in and out of the skin in this case," Nino said. Tattoo machines, depending on the number of needles attached, can make fifty to three thousand needle punctures a minute.

Yen didn't flinch as Nino repeatedly dipped the needles into the ink and worked them on her skin. "It feels like tiny little bug bites. It's a stinging sensation," she said.

Fifteen minutes after she sat down, Yen had a reddish-brown tattoo in the olive skin of her leg. Nino immediately put an antibacterial cream on the tattoo and covered it with a gauze bandage.

"In two hours," he told her, "remove the bandage and wash your skin. Don't rub it or use a washcloth. Just pat it dry with a paper towel. Put some Bacitracin or Polysporin on it and make sure you really work it into the tattoo. Keep the area clean, and keep applying the antibacterial lotion. Don't stick it out in the sun, and don't go swimming in a pool or in the ocean for at least two weeks. Saltwater, chlorine, and sun can ruin a tattoo. As it heals, you'll get a scab. That's normal. Let it heal naturally. Don't pick it."

This was all good advice. Too many people either don't get that kind of advice, or they don't follow it. Treating your skin *gently* after getting a tattoo is really important. If you don't take care of it, you can turn that tattoo into a nasty-looking blur with a permanent scar.

Rachel e-mailed that she found out the hard way: "I had a tattoo on my shoulder, and the person who did the tattoo gave me the wrong instructions for taking care of it. I was out in the sun, and I went swimming in the ocean right after. The color is muddy, and I developed an infection and an ugly scar."

There are other causes for concern as well. Nino works in a sanitary environment and uses sterile equipment. If sanitary protocols are not strictly followed, you can pick up viruses like hepatitis B or hepatitis C. Studies show that people who get tattoos are more at risk than others of being infected with hepatitis C. Many people don't discover that they have hepatitis until years after getting a tattoo, when they develop liver cancer or cirrhosis of the liver. Epidemiologists try to trace the origins of the virus, but there are many people who never connect an old tattoo to the disease.

The hepatitis viruses are spread through the blood by the use of dirty needles and dyes, which are used over and over again on many people. In some cases, the needles may start out sterile, but the tattooist may place them on a dirty surface, or jab the needles into his or her own arm to test them.

The needles can also pass on HIV, tetanus, and tuberculosis. You can protect yourself against diseases by making sure that the tattooing process is absolutely sterile.

If you have sickle-cell anemia, you're not a candidate for tattooing. Similarly, if you have a tendency to form keloids—large thick scars—tattoos are not for you. If you have allergies, or very sensitive skin, be aware that you may be allergic to the pigment in the dyes.

The technicians in any reputable tattoo parlor will ask you questions about your health before they agree to create the tattoo. They should ask if you have a blood-borne disease, or if you scar easily or form keloids. If they don't ask these questions it's a tip-off that they aren't particularly concerned with your well-being and may give you more than a tattoo.

There's one other caution. Sometimes tattoos can cause surprising medical problems. When the tattoo on Jonathan's chest suddenly started to swell, he went to see Dr. Cook-Bolden. A blood test revealed that he had a lung disease called *sarcoidosis*. "Unfortunately, the tattoo uncovered the disease, which is much more common in blacks than in others," Dr. Cook-Bolden says.

Jonathan's disease isn't life-threatening and it can be managed. Although his is an extreme case, you should be aware of all potential problems.

There are things that you can do to protect yourself against the more common problems such as infection.

What You Can Do on Your Own

Many states and cities don't regulate tattooing. And even when they do, health departments are usually too busy to make inspections, so you have to look out for your own health and safety. That's why it's important to choose your tattooist carefully. Check with the local health department and the Better Business Bureau to see if any complaints have been registered against the tattoo parlor or the artist.

When you're in the tattoo parlor, make sure it's clean. Don't be afraid to ask questions. The instruments should be cleaned in a heat and steam sterilization machine called an *autoclave*. Before the artist starts to work, make sure that he or she is using new needles that have been wrapped in a sterile package. The tattoo artist should wear a new, clean pair of gloves when working on you. And if the artist stops to do something else, like take a phone call, the gloves should be thrown away and a new pair put on.

A Doctor's Guidance

Tattoo Removal

This is a problem so many people want solved. A board-certified dermatologist or plastic surgeon who is familiar with treating skin of color and who is also a laser expert is likely to suggest removing the tattoo with an Nd:Yag laser. We describe how the laser works in chapters 19, 21, and 24. For tattoo removal, doctors should use a laser that is safe for skin of color so it won't interact negatively with your skin's pigment cells.

The laser is the best tool we have to remove tattoos, but it may not be able to remove the tattoo completely. Laser technology is constantly improving, however, and perhaps scientists will find a way to fully remove a tattoo, but we are not there yet.

In the doctor's office, you'll wear a special pair of goggles to protect your eyes. The area of the tattoo will be cleaned with antibacterial solution, and the doctor will test a small area of the tattoo to make sure you don't have a negative reaction. If your skin responds well, the doctor will zap the area repeatedly with the laser. The laser light passes through the outer layer of your skin and targets the pigment of the tattoo. The laser's heat breaks up the color in the tattoo. The tattoo pigment then scatters in tiny fragments, and those fragments are absorbed by other cells in your body.

The laser procedure can take less than five minutes, and it's likely that you'll need repeated treatments. Whether the tattoo fades or disappears depends on your skin and the colors in the tattoo. Yellows and oranges can be the most difficult colors to remove, while blue and black can be the easiest to eliminate in lighter skin types. "In skin of color," Dr. Cook-Bolden says, "blue, black, and brown can also be difficult to remove because of the close resemblance to the skin color." You may have a white patch where the tattoo was until your skin's pigment cells create new color. Dr. Downie suggests patience. "It may take many treatments over the course of a year or two before the tattoo is faded."

"Increasingly men and women are coming to my office with tattoos in the genital areas that they want removed," Dr. Downie says. "Like other tattoos these can be gradually faded. But it's rare that a tattoo can be totally removed. You're usually likely to have a small reminder."

COST

The cost of tattoo removal will vary depending on the size of the tattoo, the skill of the doctor, and where you live. Typically laser treatments for tattoo removal cost between $350 and $550 a session. You are likely to require at least twelve sessions and perhaps more than twenty to make a significant difference. Many doctors will negotiate a package price with a discount for multiple sessions.

The Bottom Line

A tattoo is a permanent mark in your skin. If you get a tattoo, make sure that it is applied in sterile, sanitary conditions. And remember, the technology is evolving, but it may be impossible to remove the tattoo completely and make your skin look the way it did before you had the permanent color applied.

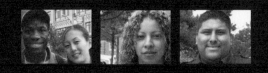

Vitiligo

CHAPTER 32

VITILIGO IS ONE OF THE MOST DISTRESSING CONDITIONS AFFLICTING skin of color. When the pigment on skin of color disappears in patches and leaves little white marks, it can be devastating. In his e-mail to us, Jared said that he felt he was disappearing: "My skin is brown and suddenly it started turning white in spots. I have white spots on my knuckles, and around my groin. There's even a white spot on my lip. I don't know how to stop this. It's scary because I'm twenty-three years old, and I'm afraid I'm going to lose all my brown color, and then I won't be me."

It is scary when vitiligo undermines your identity. And because it primarily affects people with skin of color, vitiligo is a condition that we want to cure.

Why It Happens

If we knew why it happened, we might be able to head it off. If you have vitiligo, you lose all pigment in certain areas of the skin. Doctors call this *depigmentation*. At this point, there are only theories. Vitiligo is not necessarily an inherited disease. But we think the predisposition for vitiligo is inherited. In other words, a combination of factors in your genes may

> **FACT:** *If you have vitiligo, you lose all pigment in certain areas of the skin. Doctors call this depigmentation.*

lead to the development of vitiligo, even though no one in your immediate family has it but you.

It is also possible that your immune system is at the heart of the problem, or that something in your body chemistry or your nervous system creates the climate for the pigment loss. Vitiligo is sometimes linked to thyroid disorder, anemia, diabetes, and hair loss.

Another theory is that the melanocytes, the cells that produce pigment, are destroying themselves for some reason.

Some combination of these factors may be the cause. But we just aren't certain.

FACT: *Vitiligo appears most frequently around the joints, on the fingers, wrists, and forearms, and around body openings, the lips, the eyes, genital areas, and the breasts.*

Usually, vitiligo begins at about the time that Jared noticed it. He was twenty when he began to lose pigment. We see it develop sometimes in newborns, but individuals are more likely to develop it between the ages of ten and forty.

Vitiligo appears most frequently around the joints, on the fingers, wrists, and forearms, and around body openings, the lips, the eyes, genital areas, and the breasts. Sometimes you may see a patch of white hair. Usually these white spots start out small and then morph into odd shapes.

There really is nothing that you can do on your own to stop the loss of pigment or its spread. "Trauma appears to make it worse," Dr. Cook-Bolden says. "It is very important not to rub and scratch the skin. Gentle treatment is needed here."

It's also very important to wear sun protection. Dr. Downie says, "It may sound like common sense, but it's worth saying. The darker your skin gets, the more the white spots will stand out."

If you catch the problem early, a knowledgeable doctor can help you.

Remedies

A Doctor's Guidance

First, a doctor will make sure that you have vitiligo. Doctors examine the skin using something called a Wood's Light. The doctor shines this purple, fluorescent light on the white area. If the skin looks milky white, there is a loss of pigment cells and you most likely have vitiligo. If this is verified by a biopsy of a small sample of your skin, the doctor will consider a combination of therapies.

There isn't a single remedy that works all of the time for everyone. The program that your doctor designs for you may be different from the treatment designed for another patient. It all depends on your skin, and the way it responds.

Topical steroids are usually the first line of therapy. A doctor will likely recommend a high-potency steroid that works by controlling the lymphocytes, the white blood cells, that produce a chemical that has a killing effect on the pigment cells. These potent steroids may stop the white cells from attacking the pigment. Clobex, Diprolene, Olux Foam, and Psorcon E Cream steroids are often used for this purpose.

If the vitiligo is in one or two spots, a doctor might paint a chemical called Psoralen on the skin and then expose the area to a special ultraviolet light. This therapy is called topical PUVA treatment.

For widespread vitiligo, a doctor may go further. You'll be given a Psoralen pill and required to wear protective glasses, and then you'll sit in a box fitted with ultraviolet light. The light and the Psoralen work together. PUVA treatments help to stimulate the melanocyte cells to produce color.

But one or two of these treatments is not likely to be enough. This is a big project that requires a major time commitment. You'll need about two treatments a week for months, perhaps even years, before the color returns and comes close to matching your normal skin tone.

Dr. Cook-Bolden says, "You may be surprised at what you see. As the color returns, brown dots appear in the light areas. That's because the pigment deep in our hair follicles helps to repigment the skin, and it is why it's easier to coax pigment back on hairy parts of the body."

The PUVA treatment makes eyes and skin very sensitive to sun and light. You'll have to wear goggles for several hours after you sit in the light box to prevent damage to your eyes. And when you're out in the sun, you'll have to take special precautions. Without the proper protection, your skin may get a bad burn. Sunscreens with UVA protection alone won't help. A UVA and UVB sunblock with Parsol 1789, zinc or titanium oxide, and an SPF of 30 is essential. And you'll need to wear protective clothes and a hat.

New prescription medications that work to suppress immune system may also work to treat vitiligo. Because there's the possibility that vitiligo may be the result of the immune system mistakenly producing antibodies that attack the body's own pigment cells, doctors are experimenting with drugs such as Protopic, Elidel, and Imiquimod. These drugs may stop the attack on the pigment cells. Reports are encouraging so far, particularly because these drugs appear to produce no serious side effects. Doctors are increasingly prescribing these immune modulators for treating vitiligo, although this therapy is not yet approved for this purpose by the FDA.

A new drug called Pseudocatalase is another immune system modulator. Researchers at the Northwestern University Department of Dermatology are studying its effect on vitiligo. And though

Pseudocatalase is not yet approved by the FDA, there's hope that this topical cream may be a breakthrough for treating vitiligo.

Laser Treatment

A laser using a narrow band of UVB light has been approved by the FDA for treating vitiligo. We describe how lasers work in earlier chapters. In the treatment of vitiligo, doctors direct the excimer laser at the light patches of skin to stimulate pigment. Researchers say this treatment seems to work better than other methods. Treatments are given three times a week, and some people have begun to see repigmentation after only two weeks.

COST

Laser treatments generally cost between $300 and $1,500 per session depending on the skill of the doctor and where you live. Some doctors will work out a plan to reduce the cost if you have multiple sessions.

Light Technology

ReLume Treatment

ReLume Repigmentation Phototherapy is a new system developed to treat hypopigmentation, or light spots in the skin. Although it is approved by the Food and Drug Administration for treating vitiligo, researchers are still investigating the system's effectiveness.

This nonlaser light system stimulates the melanocytes, restores pigment, and evens skin tone in some cases. ReLume works on the same principle as a tanning machine, but it is safer because it does not project ultraviolet rays.

The treatment is performed in the doctor's office. Light is applied to a specific area through a handheld device attached to a small computer that generates and regulates the light. Wavelengths of energy provoke the melanocytes to produce more color and darken the lighter spots in the target areas.

Areas where hair grows on the face, neck, and torso seem to respond better than other parts of the body. The skin on the fingers, for example, may be resistant. The number of treatments required depends on the size of the area and how the skin responds. If color does return to the skin, follow-up maintenance treatments are likely to be needed.

COST

A ReLume treatment might cost $500 to $1,000 depending on the area of the body. Because multiple sessions are required, the doctor may work out a payment program to reduce the overall cost.

Surgery

If all topical and light therapies fail, you might want to consider some type of surgery. Doctors can remove skin from one part of the body and transplant it to another part. Pigment cell transplant techniques also can be used. A surgeon will take a solution from an area of the skin with normal pigment cells, and transplant the solution in the area affected by vitiligo. When this therapy works, the solution actually becomes absorbed and the normal melanocytes produce color.

The Bottom Line

If you develop vitiligo, getting treatment early is important. There's no cure. But in many cases, treatment can make a difference. We want to encourage you to see a doctor. It's the only way to find out if you can stop the loss of pigment and put the pigment cells back to work. Treatment is long-term and requires consistent visits to the doctor's office. It may take years before you even begin to see a difference. Again, your follow-through is essential to treating the problem.

Words to the Wise

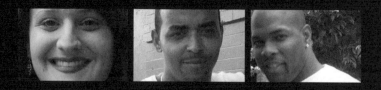

ADVANCES IN SCIENCE ARE PROVIDING NEW INSIGHT INTO THE workings of the skin and revolutionizing the way doctors approach cosmetic and medical problems. New discoveries are leading to the development of innovative ways to treat medical conditions and improve the health and the appearance of the skin. We're happy to share this information with you and we hope that you will use it *wisely*.

We've recommended many products, treatments, and remedies. Many complement each other and are best when used together or alternately in the morning and the evening. When you use our suggestions, please remember that in most cases you won't see results overnight. A consistent skin management program will help you to have healthy and beautiful skin. You can enhance every treatment by handling your skin *gently* and using the products *wisely*.

Everyone's skin reacts differently. You're the guardian of the incredible protective and beautiful barrier that nature has provided, and only you will know how your skin responds to a particular product.

People often try to clear up a problem by loading one product on top of another. They quickly discover that instead of improving their skin, they've irritated it and made an existing condition worse.

In a number of chapters we've mentioned that certain vitamins are beneficial. Vitamin A helps to stimulate the development of new collagen and renew skin cells. Vitamins C and E fight the free radicals that cause aging. Vitamin K may help to calm swollen blood vessels under the eyes. Many creams and prescription medicines contain these vitamins as well as other ingredients we've mentioned. They are effective if they are used correctly. But vitamins, products, and medicines can irritate the skin when they are overused. Ingesting huge amounts of the vitamins won't help. They may make you sick. But taking a daily multiple vitamin is an excellent idea.

Similarly, alpha and beta hydroxy acids are terrific tools that you can use at home to help renew your skin. But they too can irritate the skin if they are used incorrectly.

To use products *wisely* and carefully, we think it is a good idea to set up a simple at-home skin care management program that includes a morning and evening routine that you can follow for a long time.

Morning Care

In the morning, we suggest an alpha or beta hydroxy wash. Apply the wash *gently* and rinse with cool water. You may need a milder wash than the alpha hydroxy products can offer. NeoStrata makes cleansers with gluconolactone, which is a special formulation of alpha hydroxy acid and may be gentler on your skin. NeoStrata can be purchased via the Internet, if you can't find it in your local store.

Moisturize your body and face. We like moisturizers with sunblock and vitamins C and E. They provide a bonus. If you choose to use a retinoid in the morning, Differin is safe to use along with a sunscreen during the day when you are in the sun.

The alpha and beta hydroxy products, retinols, and hydroquinones can make your skin extremely sensitive. It is important to remember to apply sunblock repeatedly throughout the day when you're outside.

Evening Care

We suggest using retinoid products like Retin-A Micro, Avage, Tazorac, or Differin in the evening. Sunlight may interact negatively with the retinoid. If a doctor has recommended a hydroquinone product to fade dark marks and even skin color, it often works best when applied with a retinoid in the evening. In some cases, your doctor may suggest that you apply the hydroquinone twice a day.

It's possible to also use a gentle moisturizing night and eye cream. Be careful to apply everything sparingly. Let the phrase "less is more" guide you when applying all products, especially to the face.

And don't forget to moisturize your body.

Twice Daily Anti-Aging Remedies

We also suggest taking one extra step twice a day. It's a good idea to add an over-the-counter anti-aging product to your regular skin management program. Anti-aging products are effective particularly when you use them in the morning and in the evening.

There are a variety of products to choose from and they vary significantly in price. The least expensive products contain Coenzyme Q 10, an antioxidant that fights the free radicals that destroy skin cells. Most drug stores will have Eucerin Q-10 Anti-Wrinkle Sensitive Skin Cream, and Nivea's Q 10 line of products that includes Q 10 Plus Wrinkle Control, Q 10 Plus Control Night, and Plus Wrinkle Control Eye Cream.

Prevage is a more expensive topical product that's sold in doctors' offices. It contains idebenone, a chemical compound that's similar to, but more effective than, Coenzyme Q10. Idebenone has been used to treat Alzheimer patients. Now, this anti-aging, skin care formulation created by Allergan helps to protect the skin against the sun and other environmental damage. It also improves the texture of the skin, and reduces the appearance of fine lines and wrinkles.

We also like products that contain Matrixyl, a chemical compound that stimulates your natural collagen. Olay Regenerist, Alyria Revitalizing Cream, and Alyria Revitalizing Eye Serum contain Matrixyl.

Skin Medica's TNS Recovery Complex is one of our favorite anti-aging products. It contains a potent chemical compound called Nouricel-MD that combines human growth factors, soluble collagen, antioxidants that fight free radicals, and other ingredients. We like this product because it helps to even out skin pigmentation, reduces the appearance of fine lines and wrinkles, and firms up the skin. We've seen good results particularly when TNS Recovery Complex is used with a product that contains Matrixyl. TNS Recovery Complex can be purchased in doctors' offices.

When you choose an anti-aging product, it's important to use it consistently for two to three months in order to see the benefit. And remember—most anti-aging products should always be used with your regular moisturizer.

Always

Moisturizers and sunblocks are *always* your best friends. Although you may be tempted to forget them, it is *always wise* to keep a tube of moisturizer at your kitchen sink, near your desk, or where you work and to carry a tube of moisturizer and sunblock with you. Your skin can be renewed, but renewal requires effort, attention, and maintenance.

The small steps you take today can help you to *always* have healthy and beautiful skin of color.

Acknowledgments

WE ARE GRATEFUL FOR THE VISION, PERCEPTION, AND KEEN UNDER-standing of our publisher, Judith Regan. She immediately recognized the importance of providing comprehensive information about skin of color. Our profound thanks go to our editors, Aliza Fogelson, whose excellent suggestions set us on the right course, and Monica Crowley, whose wise reading and skillful editing helped to make this a book we hope you will love. We also thank our unofficial editor, Authors Guild president Nick Taylor, for his valuable guidance, enthusiasm, and patience.

Information in this book was drawn from our training, clinical experience, and many academic sources. Barbara Nevins Taylor's education was enhanced by a wide range of sources including the works of Lewis Thomas, particularly *The Lives of the Cell*, and Bryan Sykes, particularly *The Seven Daughters of Eve*. We also want to thank Nadine Tosk of the American Society for Dermatologic Surgery for providing timely information.

This book would not have been possible without the enthusiasm of the viewers of WWOR-TV, UPN9, a Fox Television Station in New York City. We appreciate their interest, support, and willingness to turn to us for information. We also wish to thank Will J. Wright, formerly news director at WWOR-TV, for encouraging Barbara Nevins Taylor to investigate issues involving skin of color. These television reports drew us together and led to our collaboration.

Attorney Gus Samios was an important voice in the early stages of the project. His good counsel is appreciated. The able research skills of Jennifer Gerardo and Joanna Cetera helped get us started and we thank you.

Dr. Cook-Bolden

My children, Natalie, Mike and Al—I thank you for open arms, kisses, and squeezes. You are the joy of my life. I wish you the best the world has to give. My husband, Michael—You are my soul mate. Thank you for keeping me on track. My mom and dad, Doris Montgomery Cook and Ralph Cook, and my sister, Tara—Your love and guidance fuel me. Thank you for your infinite wisdom. Dr. Vincent DeLeo and Reverend Rose Niles-McCrary—You have been my guiding light academically and spiritually. Minerva Rodriguez—You are my partner in patient care. Thanks for your dedication and loyalty. I thank my patients; it gives me great joy to participate in your care. I thank my friends, whose relationships mean so much in my life.

Dr. Downie

My husband, Michael Heningburg, Jr.—Thank you for your love, support, and advice. You make my life worth living. My daughter, Jade—You are my beautiful, sweet, precious girl. May your life always be filled with good luck, joy, peace, and love. My mother, Dr. Marjorie Jones—You are an inspiration. Thank you for your unconditional love and teaching me the value of hard work. My dad, Norbert Downie—You taught me to value education and the importance of negotiating skills. My brothers, Michael and Mark—I love you dearly. Dr. Patricia Wexler, Dr. Lori Polis, Dr. Alan Shalita, Dr. Raul Fleishmajer, Dr. Steven Cohen, Dr. Martin Brownstein, Dr. Cheryl Burgess, and Dr. Lynn Silverstein—thank you for being mentors and important influences in my life. Jovanna Gonzalez and the Image Dermatology staff—Thank you for helping me provide compassionate care. I thank my patients for their trust and confidence.

Disclosure

Dr. Fran Cook-Bolden is a paid consultant and researcher for the following companies:

Allergan
Andrew Jergens Company, Inc.
Dermik Laboratories
Galderma
ICN Pharmaceuticals
Lumenis
Medicis
Photonics
Roche
SkinMedica

Dr. Jeanine Downie is a paid consultant for the following companies:

Allergan
Bobbi Brown Cosmetics
Galderma
Johnson & Johnson
Merck
Parsol 1789
Palmer's Skin Success
Skin Salon Gold
Warner Chilcott

Index